ICP/API Guidelines on

Rational Prescribing Practices in the Elderly

ICP/API Guidelines on
Rational Prescribing Practices in the Elderly

Chief Advisor

RK Singal MD(General Medicine) FICP FACP(USA) FIAMS
Dean, Indian College of Physicians
Principal, Consultant and Head
Department of Internal Medicine
BLK-MAX Super Speciality Hospital
Rajinder Nagar, New Delhi, India

Editors

Jyotirmoy Pal MD FICP FRCP WHO Fellow
Professor
Department of General Medicine
Sagar Dutta Medical College and Hospital
Kolkata, West Bengal, India

Santanu K Tripathi MD DM(Clinical Pharmacology)
Former Head
Department of Clinical Pharmacology
School of Tropical Medicine
Kolkata, West Bengal, India

Arvind Mathur MD FICP
Editor, Journal of the Indian Academy of Geriatrics
Director and Managing Trustee
Asian Center for Medical Education, Research and Innovation
Chairperson, Caregivers Asha Society
Ex-Principal and Controller, Professor of Medicine
Dr Sampurnanand Medical College (SNMC)
Jodhpur, Rajasthan, India

Executive Editors

Nandini Chatterjee MBBS MD
FRCP(Glasgow) FICP
Professor
Department of Medicine
Institute of Postgraduate Medical Education
and Research (IPGMER) and SSKM Hospital
Kolkata, West Bengal, India

Shambo Samrat Samajdar MBBS MD
DM(Clinical Pharmacology)
FIPS Fellow Diabetes India PG Dip Endo and
Diabetes(RCP) Fellowship in Respiratory and
Critical Care(WBUHS) Diploma in Allergy Asthma
Immunology(BV University)
Research Wing Leader, Doctors AI
Consultant Physician, Department of General
Medicine, HealthETC
Kolkata, West Bengal, India

Under the Auspices of Indian College of Physicians,
Academic Wing of the Association of Physicians of India

JAYPEE BROTHERS MEDICAL PUBLISHERS
The Health Sciences Publisher
New Delhi | London

Jaypee Brothers Medical Publishers (P) Ltd

Headquarters
EMCA House
23/23-B, Ansari Road, Daryaganj
New Delhi 110 002, India
Landline: +91-11-23272143, +91-11-23272703
+91-11-23282021, +91-11-23245672
E-mail: jaypee@jaypeebrothers.com

Corporate Office
Jaypee Brothers Medical Publishers (P) Ltd.
4838/24, Ansari Road, Daryaganj
New Delhi 110 002, India
Phone: +91-11-43574357
Fax: +91-11-43574314
E-mail: jaypee@jaypeebrothers.com

Overseas Office
JP Medical Ltd.
83, Victoria Street, London
SW1H 0HW (UK)
Phone: +44-20 3170 8910
Fax: +44(0)20 3008 6180
E-mail: info@jpmedpub.com

Website: www.jaypeebrothers.com
Website: www.jaypeedigital.com

Inquiries for bulk sales may be solicited at: jaypee@jaypeebrothers.com

ICP/API Guidelines on Rational Prescribing Practices in the Elderly / Jyotirmoy Pal, Santanu K Tripathi, Arvind Mathur

First Edition: 2025

ISBN: 978-93-6616-690-2

Printed at: Samrat Offset Pvt. Ltd.

Advisory Board

Editorial Board

Preface

The rapid growth of the global aging population brings with it unprecedented challenges and opportunities in healthcare. As older adults increasingly live with multiple chronic conditions, often managed through complex medication regimens, the need for rational prescribing practices becomes ever more critical. The elderly population's unique physiological changes, vulnerabilities to adverse drug reactions, and frequent exposure to polypharmacy demand tailored approaches to ensuring safe, effective, and ethical medication use.

"ICP/API Guidelines on Rational Prescribing Practices in the Elderly" is designed to address these challenges comprehensively. This book provides a roadmap for healthcare professionals to navigate the complexities of prescribing for elderly patients, balancing the need for therapeutic efficacy with the imperative to minimize harm.

The chapters in this book reflect a wide range of expertise and evidence-based strategies. From understanding the physiological changes that influence drug pharmacokinetics and pharmacodynamics in aging to exploring practical tools like the Beers Criteria and STOPP/START frameworks, each section is crafted to enhance clinical decision-making. The book also delves into critical issues such as deprescribing, managing drug–drug interactions, and addressing ethical and legal considerations in elderly care.

Nonpharmacological strategies, personalized medication management, and detailed case studies further enrich the discussion, offering actionable insights into improving the quality of life for older adults. By presenting a holistic view of rational prescribing, this book aims to empower healthcare providers to adopt patient-centered approaches, foster shared decision-making, and ensure equitable, ethical, and effective care for elderly populations.

We hope this guide will serve as a valuable resource for physicians, pharmacists, nurses, and allied healthcare professionals committed to optimizing geriatric care. By combining clinical expertise, research insights, and practical tools, we strive to build a future where every elderly patient receives the best possible care, tailored to their unique needs and circumstances.

We extend our gratitude to the contributors whose efforts and expertise have shaped this comprehensive guide. May this book inspire a deeper commitment to the principles of rational prescribing and pave the way for safer, more effective healthcare practices for our aging societies.

Editorial Team
Jyotirmoy Pal
Arvind Mathur
Santanu K Tripathi
Nandini Chatterjee
Shambo Samrat Samajdar

Contents

1

CHAPTER

Rational Prescribing in the Elderly: Principles, Challenges, and Strategies for Optimizing Medication Use

ABSTRACT

Rational prescribing is a cornerstone of modern healthcare, particularly for elderly patients who face unique challenges such as polypharmacy, age-related physiological changes, and multiple chronic conditions (MCCs). This chapter provides a comprehensive overview of rational prescribing, emphasizing its importance in minimizing adverse drug reactions (ADRs), optimizing therapeutic outcomes, and enhancing quality of life. The principles of rational prescribing, including patient-centered care, evidence-based practice, and deprescribing, are explored through the 5R framework, which guides clinicians in selecting the right drug, dose, route, duration, and monitoring strategy. Special attention is given to integrating clinical pharmacology principles into elderly care through systematic approaches such as personalized dosing, collaborative decision-making, and polypharmacy management. The chapter concludes with key objectives of rational prescribing guidelines, underscoring their role in improving safety, efficacy, and patient satisfaction while addressing treatment burdens and healthcare costs.

INTRODUCTION

Prescribing medication is one of the most powerful tools available to clinicians. At its heart, the act of prescribing aims to provide tangible health benefits to patients, alleviate suffering, and enhance quality of life. However, the act of prescribing becomes significantly complex when dealing with elderly patients, particularly those with multiple chronic conditions (MCCs). For such patients, potential benefits of medication must be carefully weighed against possible harms, treatment burdens, and individual health priorities.

To understand the complexities of rational prescribing in the elderly, consider two patients with longstanding hypertension. Patient 1 is a 50-year-old woman with no other health issues, while patient 2 is an 85-year-old woman with atrial fibrillation (AF), diabetes, congestive heart failure, arthritis, and depression, each requiring its own set of medications. While the first patient can be treated with a straightforward approach focused on reducing cardiovascular risks, prescribing for the second patient requires consideration of her life expectancy, potential drug interactions, cumulative treatment burden, and her personal health goals. This chapter lays the foundation for understanding rational prescribing and its critical importance in optimizing care for the elderly population.

WHAT IS RATIONAL PRESCRIBING?

Rational prescribing is a structured approach to selecting, initiating, and monitoring medications to ensure maximum therapeutic benefit with minimal harm. It integrates scientific evidence with clinical judgment to cater to the individual needs of the patient. The World Health Organization (WHO) emphasizes that rational prescribing ensures patients receive appropriate medications for their clinical conditions in the correct doses, durations, and at the most affordable cost. This practice not only improves therapeutic outcomes but also minimizes healthcare costs and reduces the risk of adverse drug reactions (ADRs).

CORE PRINCIPLES OF RATIONAL PRESCRIBING

Appropriate Drug Selection

Medication choices must align with a thorough clinical diagnosis and consideration of patient-specific factors, such as age, existing conditions, and comorbidities. Evidence-based guidelines and drug efficacy must underpin these decisions.

Personalized Dosing

Dose adjustments are critical, especially in populations such as the elderly, where pharmacokinetics (PK) and pharmacodynamics (PD) changes can affect drug metabolism and excretion. Tailoring doses based on individual characteristics such as weight, renal function, and hepatic function is essential.

Minimization of Risks

Assessing potential risks such as ADRs, drug-drug interactions, and contraindications is fundamental. For instance, avoiding drugs with high toxicity profiles or known incompatibilities with patient conditions helps reduce harm.

Patient-centric Approach

Engaging patients in the decision-making process enhances adherence and aligns treatments with their values and preferences. This collaborative model supports shared decision-making and respects individual priorities, such as symptom management or life expectancy.

Economic Efficiency

Cost-effectiveness must be balanced with therapeutic efficacy. Choosing generic medications over branded counterparts and avoiding unnecessary polypharmacy ensures that treatments remain economically viable.

THE 5R FRAMEWORK IN RATIONAL PRESCRIBING

To operationalize rational prescribing effectively after selection of "right patient", the *5R* concept serves as a guiding framework:

1. *Right drug*: Select the drug that has proven efficacy for the condition while considering evidence from clinical trials and individual patient needs. For example, avoid prescribing broad-spectrum antibiotics unnecessarily to minimize resistance risks.
2. *Right dose*: Establish doses that achieve therapeutic outcomes while minimizing adverse effects. In the elderly, lower starting doses often mitigate risks stemming from decreased renal or hepatic function.
3. *Right route*: The administration route should optimize drug absorption and compliance. For instance, switching to oral formulations when feasible reduces complications associated with intravenous administration.
4. *Right duration*: Prescribing for the optimal duration prevents overuse or misuse. For example, limiting the duration of proton pump inhibitors (PPIs) reduces risks of osteoporosis and nutrient malabsorption.
5. *Right monitoring*: Systematic follow-up ensures therapeutic effectiveness and timely identification of side effects. For high-risk drugs, such as warfarin, regular international normalized ratio (INR) monitoring is essential to balance efficacy and safety.

IMPORTANCE OF RATIONAL PRESCRIBING IN THE ELDERLY

Older adults, often presenting with MCCs, require complex medication regimens. This population is particularly vulnerable to polypharmacy and its associated risks, including adverse drug events (ADEs), drug-drug interactions, and reduced adherence. Rational prescribing mitigates these risks by emphasizing individualized treatment plans and deprescribing unnecessary or harmful medications. By integrating the principles of rational prescribing, clinicians can enhance therapeutic outcomes, improve quality of life, and reduce healthcare costs.

RATIONAL PRESCRIBING AS AN ITERATIVE PROCESS

Rational prescribing is not static but an ongoing, patient-focused process involving:

- *Diagnosis and prognosis*: Accurate diagnosis and a realistic understanding of patient prognosis guide medication decisions.
- *Treatment goals*: Establish clear objectives, such as symptom relief, disease modification, or prevention of complications.
- *Therapeutic trials*: Conduct controlled medication trials to assess efficacy and safety, particularly in cases involving complex drug regimens.
- *Patient engagement*: Involve patients in defining goals and understanding trade-offs, fostering adherence, and satisfaction.

Rational prescribing is a cornerstone of modern medicine that demands a balance of evidence, clinical expertise, and patient-centric care. By adhering to the principles and the 5R framework, healthcare providers can ensure medications are used responsibly and effectively, particularly in vulnerable populations such as the elderly.

IMPORTANCE OF RATIONAL PRESCRIBING IN THE ELDERLY

Elderly patients present unique challenges for prescribing due to age-related physiological changes, polypharmacy, and the prevalence of MCCs. These factors significantly increase the risks of ADEs, treatment burdens, and reduced quality of life. A rational prescribing approach becomes critical to navigate these complexities and optimize care outcomes.

Key Challenges in the Elderly

Polypharmacy

Defined as the concurrent use of five or more medications, polypharmacy is prevalent among elderly patients due to the need to manage multiple chronic diseases such as diabetes, hypertension, and osteoarthritis. However, polypharmacy increases the likelihood of ADRs, drug-drug interactions, and prescribing cascades, ultimately impairing adherence.

Studies reveal that nearly half of elderly individuals take more than five medications daily, with many facing complications such as cognitive decline, frailty, and falls due to improper medication management.

Age-related Physiological Changes

The elderly experience significant PK and PD changes, impacting drug absorption, distribution, metabolism, and elimination:

- *Reduced metabolism*: Decreased hepatic enzyme activity, particularly in Phase I metabolic pathways, prolongs drug half-lives (e.g., benzodiazepines).
- *Impaired excretion*: Declining renal function (lowered glomerular filtration rates) impacts drug clearance, necessitating dose adjustments for renally excreted drugs such as digoxin and aminoglycosides.

Such changes often lead to enhanced drug sensitivity, especially for central nervous system (CNS)-active agents, increasing risks of sedation and delirium.

Drug-disease Interactions

Many drugs exacerbate preexisting conditions in the elderly:

- Anticholinergics can worsen dementia symptoms by impairing cognition.
- Nonsteroidal anti-inflammatory drugs (NSAIDs) exacerbate hypertension and can lead to renal impairment.

Treatment Burden

Complex medication regimens impose cognitive and physical demands, reducing adherence, and increasing risks of hospitalizations. Elderly individuals often report difficulties managing polypharmacy, compounded by the logistical and financial barriers to accessing healthcare.

BENEFITS OF RATIONAL PRESCRIBING FOR ELDERLY PATIENTS

Rational prescribing is a patient-centered approach that enhances safety and optimizes therapeutic outcomes, ensuring alignment with the patient's health priorities.

- *Enhancing safety*:
    - Proactive deprescribing minimizes ADEs, particularly those arising from inappropriate medication use.
    - Tools such as the STOPP/START criteria and Beers List help identify high-risk medications, such as benzodiazepines and anticholinergics, which are common culprits of ADRs in the elderly.
- *Improving outcomes*: Rational prescribing ensures medications achieve intended therapeutic goals while respecting the patient's unique physiological profile, e.g., adjusting antihypertensive therapies for frail elderly individuals to prevent falls caused by orthostatic hypotension.
- *Reducing costs*: Preventing ADEs and hospitalizations reduces healthcare costs. Rational deprescribing of statins in end-of-life care, e.g., is both cost-effective and improves quality of life.
- *Promoting deprescribing*: A systematic review of the patient's medication regimen helps to discontinue unnecessary or potentially harmful drugs, reducing treatment burden, and improving adherence. Tools like the "Brown Bag Medication Review" facilitate accurate reconciliation.

PRINCIPLES OF SAFE AND EFFECTIVE PRESCRIBING

Rational prescribing is guided by several foundational principles that prioritize patient safety, efficacy, and individualized care.

Patient-centered Care

Prioritize the patient's health goals, values, and preferences during decision-making. Engage in shared discussions to ensure adherence and satisfaction.

Evidence-based Practice

Use clinical guidelines, research evidence, and expert consensus to inform prescribing decisions. Be cautious when extrapolating data from younger populations to elderly patients.

Comprehensive Assessment

Evaluate the patient's clinical history, medication use, renal and hepatic function, and other factors that influence drug safety and efficacy.

Deprescribing

Regularly review and discontinue medications that are no longer necessary, ineffective, or harmful.

Minimizing Polypharmacy

Avoid prescribing unnecessary medications. Focus on the most effective treatments with minimal risk.

Monitoring and Follow-up

Continuously assess the effectiveness and safety of prescribed medications. Be vigilant for ADRs, drug interactions, and changes in clinical status.

Risk-benefit Analysis

Balance the potential benefits of treatment against the risks, considering the patient's life expectancy and health priorities.

Education and Communication

Provide clear instructions to patients and caregivers regarding medication use, potential side effects, and adherence strategies.

COMPREHENSIVE INTEGRATION OF CLINICAL PHARMACOLOGY PRINCIPLES INTO ELDERLY CARE

The *Clinical Pharmacological Reconciliation, Review, and Feedback (CPRRF)* framework has emerged as a transformative approach to improving elderly care. This method aims to optimize prescribing practices by integrating personalized and evidence-based pharmacological principles. A detailed, 10-step framework is presented here, expanding upon the CPRRF methodology for rational prescribing in elderly populations.

1. Medication Necessity Evaluation

- *Description*: Regularly assess the necessity of each medication in the context of the patient's current clinical status, ensuring alignment with therapeutic goals.
- *Objective*: Avoid unnecessary or duplicative prescriptions that contribute to polypharmacy.
- *Implementation*: Review each prescription's purpose during consultations and healthcare transitions.

2. Deprescribing Practices

- *Description*: Proactively identify and discontinue medications with no therapeutic benefit or those posing significant harm.
- *Objective*: Reduce polypharmacy and ADRs while improving quality of life.
- *Implementation*: Use structured tools like the STOPP/START criteria and Beers Criteria to identify inappropriate medications.

3. Transitional Care Optimization

- *Description*: Ensure medication continuity and accuracy during transitions between healthcare settings, such as hospital discharge to home care.

- *Objective*: Prevent medication errors and adverse outcomes during transitions.
- *Implementation*: Employ standardized medication reconciliation processes during every transition phase.

4. Personalized Dosing

- *Description*: Adjust drug dosages to accommodate the unique PK and PD of elderly patients.
- *Objective*: Achieve optimal therapeutic outcomes while minimizing side effects.
- *Implementation*: Consider renal and hepatic function, body composition changes, and drug metabolism rates when determining doses.

5. Adverse Reaction Identification and Management

- *Description*: Monitor for and address ADRs promptly to prevent exacerbation of health conditions or reduced treatment adherence.
- *Objective*: Sustain a safe and effective pharmacological regimen.
- *Implementation*: Encourage caregivers to report potential ADRs and use technology solutions for real-time monitoring.

6. Polypharmacy Rationalization

- *Description*: Streamline medication regimens to reduce drug-drug and drug-disease interactions.
- *Objective*: Minimize risks associated with cumulative pharmacological effects.
- *Implementation*: Regularly review and consolidate treatment plans through interdisciplinary collaboration.

7. Comprehensive Monitoring

- *Description*: Conduct regular follow-ups to evaluate the ongoing effectiveness of prescribed medications.
- *Objective*: Ensure treatment regimens remain aligned with the patient's evolving health needs and priorities.
- *Implementation*: Incorporate tools such as therapeutic drug monitoring (TDM) and patient-reported outcomes.

8. Collaborative Decision-making

- *Description*: Engage patients and caregivers in shared discussions regarding treatment plans, emphasizing their preferences and goals.
- *Objective*: Foster adherence and satisfaction while maintaining patient autonomy.
- *Implementation*: Utilize tools like SMART (Specific, Measurable, Achievable, Relevant, Time-bound) goals to define clear therapeutic objectives.

9. Accessibility and Affordability

- *Description*: Address economic and logistical barriers to medication adherence, ensuring treatments are within the patient's financial means.

- *Objective*: Promote equitable access to essential therapies without undue burden.
- *Implementation*: Provide generic alternatives and leverage governmental or community health support programs.

10. Enhancing Quality of Life

- *Description*: Tailor interventions to prioritize the overall well-being and dignity of elderly patients, beyond mere disease management.
- *Objective*: Shift the focus from survival metrics to a more holistic view of patient satisfaction and independence.
- *Implementation*: Emphasize nonpharmacological interventions, such as physical therapy and dietary modifications, as complementary to pharmacological care.

IMPACT AND FUTURE DIRECTIONS

The CPRRF framework enhances the safety and efficacy of medication management in elderly patients. By addressing the multidimensional challenges of aging, including polypharmacy, altered PK/PD responses, and the psychosocial needs of patients, this approach lays the foundation for more empathetic and effective elderly care.

Through systematic adoption and refinement, the CPRRF principles hold promise for transforming elderly care into a model of precision, collaboration, and respect, ultimately improving health outcomes and patient satisfaction.

Table 1 outlines the steps and key considerations in rational prescribing for elderly patients, providing a structured framework for clinicians to optimize medication use in this population. Beginning with the accurate diagnosis of presenting symptoms, past medical history, and investigations, the process incorporates patient-centered approaches by aligning treatment options with individual expectations, values, and goals such as symptom control or quality of life improvement. Prescribing involves careful selection of drug, dose, route, and duration, guided by PK, PD, evidence, and cost-effectiveness. Patient-specific factors, including age, sex, coexisting diseases, and genetic influences, are considered to ensure safety and efficacy. Comprehensive patient counseling clarifies the rationale, expected effects, and potential adverse reactions of the prescribed therapy. Finally, regular monitoring and follow-up assess therapeutic outcomes, adherence, and the need for adjustments, ensuring a dynamic and responsive approach to treatment in elderly patients.

OBJECTIVES OF RATIONAL PRESCRIBING GUIDELINES

The guidelines aim to equip healthcare providers with tools and strategies to enhance prescribing practices, particularly for elderly patients with MCCs. Key objectives include:

- *Improving safety*: Reduce the incidence of ADRs, medication errors, and inappropriate prescribing.
- *Enhancing efficacy*: Ensure prescribed medications effectively address the patient's conditions and health priorities.

TABLE 1: Steps and key considerations in rational prescribing for elderly patients.

Step	Subcomponents	Key considerations
1. Making the diagnosis	Presenting symptoms	Identify presenting symptoms, past medical and drug history, and relevant examination findings and investigations
	Past medical history and drug history	
	Examination findings	
	Investigations	
2. Consideration of treatment options	Patient wishes and expectations	Align treatment with patient's expectations, values, and prognosis, focusing on goals (e.g., cure and prevention)
	Goals of therapy	Include objectives such as symptom control, quality of life, and prevention of progression
3. Prescription	Drug, dose, route, frequency, and duration	Balance pharmacokinetics, pharmacodynamics, evidence base, and cost-effectiveness for optimal medication selection
4. Patient factors	Age and sex	Evaluate patient-specific variables such as age, sex, coexisting diseases, and genetic influences
	Interacting diseases	
	Interactive drugs	
	Genetics	
5. Patient counseling	Explanation of the prescription	Educate the patient about the rationale, expected effects, and possible adverse effects of the prescribed therapy
6. Monitoring	Monitoring effects and follow-up	Ensure close follow-up to evaluate treatment effects, compliance, and the need for any adjustments

- *Promoting deprescribing*: Systematically discontinue medications that no longer provide significant benefit or pose undue risks.
- *Addressing polypharmacy*: Minimize the use of unnecessary medications, focusing on those that are essential for achieving therapeutic goals.
- *Tailoring care*: Adapt drug regimens to the patient's age, comorbidities, and functional status.
- *Reducing treatment burden*: Simplify medication regimens and use nonpharmacologic interventions wherever feasible.
- *Cost-effectiveness*: Prescribe cost-effective treatments to reduce financial strain on patients and the healthcare system.
- *Enhancing patient involvement*: Empower patients to participate actively in their care by aligning treatments with their goals and preferences.
- *Encouraging regular reviews*: Advocate for periodic medication reviews to reassess the appropriateness and necessity of each drug.
- *Promoting healthcare coordination*: Foster collaboration among healthcare providers to streamline care and avoid fragmented or redundant treatments.

Box 1 provides a comprehensive framework for rational prescribing in the elderly, emphasizing patient-centered care, and evidence-based practices. It highlights key strategies such as prioritizing patient goals, minimizing

BOX 1 Comprehensive recommendations for rational prescribing in the elderly.

- *Prioritize patient goals*: Tailor medication plans to align with individual health priorities and life objectives
- *Evidence-based prescribing*: Use established guidelines and clinical evidence to inform treatment choices, ensuring safety, and efficacy
- *Regular medication reconciliation*: Continuously review medications to identify and remove unnecessary or duplicative prescriptions
- *Account for pharmacokinetics and pharmacodynamics changes*: Adjust dosages based on age-related physiological changes, such as reduced renal or hepatic function
- *Avoid prescribing cascades*: Address underlying causes of symptoms rather than adding medications to manage side effects
- *Minimize polypharmacy*: Limit the use of multiple medications unless clearly indicated by clinical necessity
- *Use STOPP/START criteria*: Employ these tools to identify inappropriate or essential medications in elderly patients
- *Simplify medication regimens*: Opt for straightforward dosing schedules to enhance adherence and reduce cognitive burden
- *Engage clinical pharmacology outpatient departments (OPDs)*: Collaborate with medical professionals trained in clinical pharmacology to conduct comprehensive medication reviews and provide recommendations
- *Proactive deprescribing*: Identify and discontinue medications that are no longer beneficial or pose significant risks
- *Shared decision-making*: Collaborate with patients and caregivers to explain deprescribing and engage them in medication decisions
- *Gradual tapering*: Discontinue medications systematically to prevent withdrawal effects or symptom recurrence
- *Personalized dosing*: Tailor drug dosages based on renal and hepatic function, body weight, and other individual factors
- *Start low and go slow*: Use the lowest effective dose initially, especially for CNS-active medications, to minimize adverse effects
- *Monitor for adverse drug reactions (ADRs)*: Conduct regular assessments for ADRs, drug interactions, and drug-disease conflicts
- *Avoid high-risk medications*: Refrain from prescribing benzodiazepines, anticholinergics, and nonsteroidal anti-inflammatory drugs (NSAIDs) in high-risk elderly populations
- *Opt for nonpharmacologic interventions*: Consider physical therapy, cognitive-behavioral therapy, or lifestyle modifications before initiating medications
- *Simplify dosing schedules*: Prefer once-daily regimens to enhance compliance and reduce complexity
- *Patient and caregiver education*: Provide clear and accessible instructions on medication use, potential side effects, and the importance of adherence
- *Therapeutic drug monitoring*: Regularly monitor high-risk drugs, such as anticoagulants, to ensure efficacy and minimize complications
- *Assess drug-disease interactions*: Adjust treatment regimens to prevent medications from exacerbating chronic conditions
- *Address cognitive impairments*: Avoid medications like anticholinergics that worsen cognitive function and involve caregivers in the management plan
- *Tailor antihypertensive therapy*: Adjust regimens for conditions like orthostatic hypotension to reduce fall risks in elderly patients
- *Optimize anticoagulation therapy*: Replace warfarin with direct oral anticoagulants (DOACs) when appropriate to minimize monitoring burdens and reduce bleeding risks

Continued

Continued

- *Limit long-term proton pump inhibitor (PPI) use*: Avoid prolonged PPI therapy unless necessary, to prevent complications like osteoporosis
- *Prescribe safer antidepressants*: Opt for nonsedating selective serotonin reuptake inhibitors (SSRIs) instead of tricyclics for managing depression in elderly patients
- *Address insomnia with nonpharmacologic options*: Prioritize sleep hygiene and behavioral interventions before using sedatives
- *Reassess chronic medications regularly*: Align ongoing prescriptions with the patient's current clinical status and goals
- *Promote quality of life*: Focus on improving functionality, independence, and symptom management rather than aggressive treatment
- *Avoid aggressive treatments in end-of-life care*: Refrain from life-prolonging interventions with minimal benefit for patients nearing the end of life
- *Leverage decision-support tools*: Utilize electronic systems and guidelines to enhance accuracy and identify risks in prescribing
- *Enhance safety for frail patients*: Avoid drugs with high risks of sedation, falls, or cognitive impairment
- *Involve families in decision-making*: Include caregivers in discussions about medication plans and adherence strategies
- *Promote adherence*: Reinforce the importance of following prescribed regimens during counseling sessions
- *Reduce treatment burden*: Simplify regimens and use combination therapies when possible to minimize physical and cognitive strain
- *Educate healthcare providers*: Provide regular training for clinicians on geriatric clinical pharmacology and rational prescribing practices
- *Utilize technology*: Employ electronic health records and prescribing software to improve medication management and safety
- *Address accessibility and affordability*: Prescribe cost-effective medications and leverage community support programs to ensure access
- *Employ transitional care strategies*: Conduct medication reconciliation during care transitions to prevent errors and ensure continuity
- *Set SMART therapeutic goals*: Establish specific, measurable, achievable, relevant, and time-bound objectives to guide treatment outcomes

polypharmacy, and leveraging tools like STOPP/START criteria to optimize medication safety and efficacy. Recommendations focus on simplifying regimens, engaging caregivers, and incorporating regular monitoring to address age-related physiological changes and reduce treatment burdens. This approach ensures tailored, safe, and effective medication use, enhancing therapeutic outcomes and quality of life for elderly patients.

CONCLUSION

Rational prescribing in the elderly is a complex yet essential aspect of modern healthcare. The unique challenges posed by age-related physiological changes, polypharmacy, and MCCs necessitate a thoughtful and patient-centered approach to medication management. By adhering to evidence-based principles and leveraging frameworks such as the 5R concept, clinicians can ensure optimal therapeutic outcomes while minimizing risks and burdens for elderly patients.

This chapter highlights the critical role of rational prescribing in addressing safety, efficacy, and cost-effectiveness, emphasizing the importance of tailoring treatment plans to individual patient needs and preferences. Through regular medication reviews, collaborative decision-making, and proactive deprescribing, healthcare providers can optimize care delivery, reduce ADRs, and enhance the quality of life for elderly individuals. The adoption of these practices not only improves outcomes for patients but also promotes sustainable healthcare systems, making rational prescribing a vital component of geriatric medicine.

CASE 1: POLYPHARMACY MANAGEMENT IN AN ELDERLY PATIENT WITH MULTIPLE CHRONIC CONDITIONS

Patient Background

Mr A is an 82-year-old male with a medical history of type 2 diabetes, hypertension, chronic kidney disease (stage 3), osteoarthritis, and mild cognitive impairment. He takes eight medications daily, including metformin, losartan, furosemide, atorvastatin, paracetamol, omeprazole, aspirin, and a multivitamin.

Clinical Challenge

Mr A presents to the clinic with complaints of fatigue, dizziness, and occasional confusion. His daughter expresses concern about his adherence to medications, as he often forgets which pills to take.

Rational Prescribing Approach

Diagnosis and Medication Reconciliation

Confirmed medication adherence issues and side effects, including potential over-diuresis from furosemide and polypharmacy contributing to confusion.

Blood tests revealed mild hyponatremia likely related to furosemide use.

Assessment of Goals and Priorities

- Mr A prioritizes reducing dizziness and fatigue to remain active and independent.
- Agrees to simplify the regimen while maintaining essential treatments.

Deprescribing and Tailoring Therapy

- Discontinued omeprazole and multivitamin after confirming no ongoing indications.
- Reduced furosemide dosage with regular monitoring of weight and edema.
- Simplified paracetamol dosing to as-needed for osteoarthritis pain.

Monitoring and Follow-up

- Scheduled a follow-up in 2 weeks to evaluate dizziness and electrolyte levels.
- Engaged Mr A and his daughter in medication education to improve adherence.

Outcome

After 2 weeks, Mr A reported significant improvement in symptoms. The reduced medication burden enhanced his adherence, and laboratory tests showed corrected hyponatremia.

CASE 2: ADDRESSING ADVERSE DRUG REACTIONS IN AN ELDERLY PATIENT WITH DEPRESSION AND HYPERTENSION

Patient Background

Mrs B is a 79-year-old female with a history of hypertension, depression, and insomnia. Her medications include sertraline, amlodipine, zolpidem, and over-the-counter herbal supplements.

Clinical Challenge

Mrs B reports excessive daytime drowsiness, frequent falls, and worsening memory. Her family is concerned about her safety and declining cognitive function.

Rational Prescribing Approach

Comprehensive Review

- Identified zolpidem as a probable cause of daytime sedation and increased fall risk.
- Assessed for drug-disease interactions, particularly the potential exacerbation of cognitive impairment by sedative use.

Shared Decision-making

- Discussed the risks of continuing zolpidem and proposed alternative strategies for managing insomnia.
- Mrs B agreed to taper off zolpidem gradually while exploring nonpharmacologic options.

Medication Adjustment

- Discontinued zolpidem over two weeks with a sleep hygiene plan, including cognitive behavioral therapy for insomnia (CBT-I).
- Optimized sertraline dosing for depression management without sedative effects.

Monitoring

Arranged biweekly check-ins to assess sleep patterns, mood, and cognitive function.

Outcome

Mrs B's daytime drowsiness and fall episodes resolved. She reported improved sleep quality with behavioral therapy and her family noted enhanced cognitive clarity.

CASE 3: OPTIMIZING ANTICOAGULATION IN AN ELDERLY PATIENT WITH ATRIAL FIBRILLATION AND FRAILTY

Patient Background

Mr C is an 86-year-old male with nonvalvular AF, a history of gastrointestinal bleeding, and frailty. He is currently on warfarin for stroke prevention.

Clinical Challenge

Mr C presents with recurrent bruising and concerns about frequent blood draws for INR monitoring, which he finds burdensome due to mobility issues.

Rational Prescribing Approach

Evaluation

Reviewed bleeding history and INR trends, revealing unstable control with recent values above the therapeutic range.

Discussed risks and benefits of continuing warfarin versus switching to a direct oral anticoagulant (DOAC).

Patient-centered Goals

Mr C prioritized reducing the burden of frequent monitoring and minimizing bleeding risks.

Therapeutic Adjustment

Transitioned from warfarin to apixaban, a DOAC with a favorable safety profile for elderly patients and reduced bleeding risk.

Education and Monitoring

- Provided education on DOAC use, emphasizing adherence, and recognizing signs of bleeding.
- Scheduled follow-ups every three months to monitor renal function and ensure therapeutic appropriateness.

Outcome

Mr C reported relief from the logistical challenges of INR monitoring and experienced no new bleeding episodes. His overall satisfaction and quality of life improved.

These cases highlight the application of rational prescribing principles in diverse clinical scenarios involving elderly patients. By addressing challenges such as polypharmacy, ADRs, and treatment burdens, these examples illustrate how personalized, evidence-based approaches can optimize therapeutic outcomes and enhance the quality of life in this vulnerable population.

SUGGESTED READINGS

1. Maxwell SR. Rational prescribing: the principles of drug selection. Clin Med (Lond). 2016;16(5):459-64.
2. Ouellet GM, Ouellet JA, Tinetti ME. Principle of rational prescribing and deprescribing in older adults with multiple chronic conditions. Ther Adv Drug Saf. 2018;9(11):639-52.
3. Samajdar SS, Mukherjee S, Sharma J, Pal J, Tripathi SK, Saboo B, et al. Clinical Pharmacological Reconciliation, Review, and Feedback in Elderly Care: A Transformative Approach. J Indian Acad Geriatr. 2024;20(3):150-3.
4. Samajdar SS, Tripathi SK. Clinical Pharmacological Reconciliation, Review, and Feedback in Ensuring Patient Safety: A Commentary. J Clin Pharmacol. 2023;63(9):1074-5.

2

CHAPTER

Age-related Physiological and Pharmacokinetic–Pharmacodynamic Changes

ABSTRACT

Aging is associated with progressive physiological changes across various body systems, influencing pharmacokinetics and pharmacodynamics. These changes alter drug absorption, distribution, metabolism, and excretion while modifying receptor sensitivity and homeostatic regulation. In the elderly, these factors elevate the risk of adverse drug events (ADEs) and therapeutic inefficacy. This chapter provides an in-depth analysis of age-related changes in key physiological systems, emphasizing their clinical implications and practical management strategies. Highlighted are the impacts on the nervous, cardiovascular, respiratory, gastrointestinal, musculoskeletal, endocrine, and renal systems, with tailored recommendations for rational prescribing. Through illustrative case scenarios, the chapter offers actionable insights for optimizing therapeutic outcomes while minimizing ADEs in the elderly.

INTRODUCTION

The process of aging entails a series of complex physiological changes that affect multiple systems in the human body. These changes impact functional capacity, resilience to environmental stressors, and susceptibility to diseases. In clinical practice, these physiological shifts significantly influence how elderly patients respond to medications. The altered pharmacodynamic (PD) and pharmacokinetic (PK) profiles necessitate tailored prescribing strategies to ensure efficacy and safety.

This chapter examines age-related changes in key body systems and their pharmacological implications. By understanding these changes, clinicians can adopt evidence-based prescribing practices, minimize the risks of ADEs, and address the unique needs of the elderly. The chapter integrates detailed insights into physiological alterations, pharmacological adjustments, and practical scenarios to bridge the gap between theory and clinical practice.

Aging is characterized by progressive and cumulative physiological changes across various systems in the body. These changes impact an individual's functional capacity, ability to adapt to environmental stressors, and susceptibility to diseases. The following is a detailed analysis of the age-related changes in key physiological systems.

NERVOUS SYSTEM

Aging significantly affects the nervous system leading to structural and functional changes that impair cognition, motor skills, and sensory perception. **Table 1** outlines the key age-related physiological changes in the nervous system, highlighting their specific impacts on memory, mood, coordination, and overall neurological health.

Key Changes

- *Neuron loss:* Gradual loss of neurons in the brain and spinal cord affects signal transmission.
- *Reduced neurotransmitter levels:* Decline in dopamine, serotonin, and acetylcholine contributes to slower reaction times, mood changes, and memory impairment.
- *Cerebral atrophy:* Reduction in brain volume, especially in the hippocampus and cortex, impairs memory and executive function
- *Slower reflexes:* Decreased speed of signal transmission affects motor responses and balance.

Clinical Implications

- Increased risk of neurodegenerative diseases (e.g., Alzheimer's, Parkinson's)
- Slower cognitive processing and impaired coordination
- Higher susceptibility to falls and injuries due to diminished reflexes

CARDIOVASCULAR SYSTEM

The cardiovascular system undergoes structural and functional deterioration with age, increasing the risk of cardiovascular diseases. **Table 2** summarizes the physiological changes in the cardiovascular system due to aging, emphasizing their effects on heart function, blood pressure (BP) regulation, and vascular health.

Key Changes

- *Reduced cardiac output:* A decline in heart muscle elasticity and contractility reduces pumping efficiency.

TABLE 1: Age-related changes in nervous system function and their clinical impact.

Parameter	Age-related change	Impact
Neurotransmitters	Reduced dopamine and serotonin levels	Memory loss, mood changes, and slower reflexes
Hippocampus volume	Shrinkage	Impaired learning and memory retention
Motor neuron efficiency	Decline	Poor coordination and increased fall risk

TABLE 2: Cardiovascular system changes with aging and their clinical implications.

Parameter	Age-related change	Impact
Heart elasticity	Decrease	Reduced pumping efficiency
Arterial compliance	Stiffening	Hypertension and increased cardiovascular workload
Baroreceptor sensitivity	Decrease	Orthostatic hypotension and dizziness

TABLE 3: Respiratory system alterations in aging and their effects.

Parameter	Age-related change	Impact
Lung compliance	Reduced elasticity	Decreased vital capacity and exercise tolerance
Alveolar surface area	Decreased	Impaired gas exchange and lower oxygen levels
Respiratory muscles	Weakness	Difficulty in deep breathing

- *Vascular stiffness:* Thickening and stiffening of arterial walls increase BP.
- *Reduced baroreceptor sensitivity:* Impaired regulation of BP leads to orthostatic hypotension.
- *Increased peripheral resistance:* Reduced arterial compliance contributes to systemic hypertension.

Clinical Implications

- Higher risk of hypertension, atherosclerosis, and heart failure
- Reduced exercise tolerance and slower recovery from physical exertion
- Increased risk of postural dizziness and falls

RESPIRATORY SYSTEM

Aging impacts the respiratory system's structure and function, reducing lung capacity and gas exchange efficiency. **Table 3** highlights the key respiratory system changes associated with aging, detailing their impacts on lung function, gas exchange efficiency, and breathing capacity.

Key Changes

- *Decreased lung elasticity:* Loss of elastin fibers leads to reduced lung compliance.
- *Weakened respiratory muscles:* Diaphragm and intercostal muscles lose strength, limiting airflow.
- *Decline in alveolar surface area* reduces gas exchange capacity.
- *Impaired ciliary function* hinders mucus clearance, increasing infection risk.

Clinical Implications

- Reduced ability to tolerate physical activity
- Increased risk of respiratory infections, such as pneumonia
- Decreased oxygenation during exertion

GASTROINTESTINAL SYSTEM

Aging affects the gastrointestinal (GI) system's motility, secretion, and absorption functions. **Table 4** describes the physiological changes in the GI system with aging, focusing on their effects on digestion, nutrient absorption, and GI health.

Key Changes

- *Slowed peristalsis:* Reduced muscle tone leads to slower bowel movements.
- *Reduced gastric acid secretion:* Decreases nutrient absorption, particularly calcium, iron, and vitamin B12
- *Atrophic gastric mucosa:* Increased risk of GI discomfort and infections
- *Weakened sphincters:* Increased risk of gastroesophageal reflux disease (GERD)

Clinical Implications

- Increased risk of constipation and nutrient deficiencies
- Higher susceptibility to acid reflux and gastritis
- Reduced tolerance to certain medications due to altered metabolism

MUSCULOSKELETAL SYSTEM

The musculoskeletal system undergoes structural degeneration, reducing strength, mobility, and independence. **Table 5** outlines the primary age-related changes in the musculoskeletal system, emphasizing their effects on bone health, muscle strength, and joint functionality.

Key Changes

- *Loss of bone density:* Accelerates after menopause in women, increasing fracture risk
- *Sarcopenia:* Progressive muscle mass loss leads to weakness and frailty
- *Joint degeneration:* Cartilage erosion and stiffening reduce joint mobility

TABLE 4: Age-related changes in gastrointestinal function and their clinical impact

Parameter	Age-related change	Impact
Peristalsis	Slower	Constipation and increased transit time
Gastric acid production	Decrease	Impaired nutrient absorption
Sphincter strength	Weakening	Increased risk of GERD

(GERD: gastroesophageal reflux disease)

TABLE 5: Musculoskeletal system changes with aging and their implications.

Parameter	Age-related change	Impact
Bone density	Reduction	Increased fracture risk
Muscle mass	Decline due to sarcopenia	Weakness and reduced mobility
Joint cartilage	Degeneration	Stiffness and joint pain

Clinical Implications

- Higher risk of falls, fractures, and osteoarthritis
- Reduced physical activity and independence
- Increased disability and dependency on daily activities

ENDOCRINE SYSTEM

Aging alters hormonal regulation, affecting metabolism, growth, and homeostasis. **Table 6** highlights the significant endocrine changes associated with aging, focusing on their impact on metabolism, muscle and fat composition, and bone health.

Key Changes

- *Reduced growth hormone:* Leads to loss of lean body mass and increased fat mass
- *Decline in sex hormones:* Reduced estrogen and testosterone levels impact bone density and muscle mass.
- *Impaired glucose regulation:* Decreased insulin sensitivity raises the risk of type 2 diabetes.
- *Thyroid function changes:* Subtle alterations in thyroid hormone levels may affect metabolic rate.

Clinical Implications

- Increased prevalence of osteoporosis and sarcopenia
- Higher risk of metabolic syndrome and diabetes
- Suboptimal adaptation to stress and energy demands

RENAL AND URINARY SYSTEM

Aging affects renal function, compromising the body's ability to regulate fluid and electrolyte balance. **Table 7** summarizes the physiological changes in the renal

TABLE 6: Endocrine system changes in aging and their clinical effects.

Parameter	Age-related change	Impact
Growth hormone	Decline	Loss of muscle and increased fat mass
Insulin sensitivity	Reduced	Increased risk of type 2 diabetes
Sex hormones	Decreased	Bone loss and reduced muscle mass

TABLE 7: Renal and urinary system alterations with aging and their effects.

Parameter	Age-related change	Impact
GFR	Decline	Reduced drug clearance and waste excretion
Bladder elasticity	Loss of tone	Increased urinary urgency and incontinence
Renal blood flow	Decrease	Impaired kidney function

(GFR: glomerular filtration rate)

and urinary systems due to aging, detailing their impact on kidney function, waste excretion, and urinary control.

Key Changes

- *Reduced glomerular filtration rate (GFR):* Declines by up to 50% by age 80
- *Loss of nephrons:* Reduces kidney filtering capacity
- *Decreased renal blood flow:* Limits nutrient and oxygen supply to the kidneys
- *Bladder elasticity decline:* Leads to urinary urgency and incontinence

Clinical Implications

- Altered drug clearance, necessitating dose adjustments
- Increased risk of dehydration and electrolyte imbalance
- Higher prevalence of urinary incontinence and infections

Age-related physiological changes affect all major systems in the body, leading to increased vulnerability to diseases and functional impairments. A thorough understanding of these changes is crucial for developing targeted strategies to mitigate their effects and improve the quality of life for the elderly population. Effective interventions include lifestyle modifications, pharmacological adjustments, and regular monitoring of health parameters.

CLINICAL CASE SCENARIOS: PRACTICAL IMPLICATIONS OF AGE-RELATED PHYSIOLOGICAL CHANGES

Case 1: Impaired Drug Clearance and Renal Function

Background

Mrs S, a 78-year-old woman with a history of hypertension and type 2 diabetes, presents with confusion, reduced urine output, and mild swelling in her legs. She was recently prescribed a nonsteroidal anti-inflammatory drug (NSAID) for knee pain.

Discussion

Mrs S's symptoms highlight age-related changes in renal function:

- *Key changes in renal system*:
  - Declined GFR has reduced her ability to clear renally excreted drugs.
  - NSAIDs impair renal perfusion by inhibiting prostaglandins, exacerbating her renal insufficiency.
  - Loss of nephron functionality and decreased renal blood flow increase her susceptibility to acute kidney injury.

Management

- Discontinue NSAIDs and start a kidney-friendly analgesic such as acetaminophen.
- Monitor renal function through creatinine clearance and GFR.
- Adjust antihypertensive medications as necessary to avoid further renal damage.

Clinical Pearls

- Renal insufficiency in the elderly necessitates careful selection and dose adjustment of renally excreted drugs.
- Regular monitoring of renal parameters is crucial to prevent drug-induced nephrotoxicity.

Case 2: Cardiovascular Complications and Baroreceptor Sensitivity

Background

Mr R, an 82-year-old man, presents to the emergency department after experiencing dizziness and a fall. He reports feeling lightheaded when standing and has a history of hypertension managed with a beta-blocker and diuretic.

Discussion

Mr R's presentation underscores cardiovascular system changes due to aging:

- *Key changes in cardiovascular system*:
    - Reduced *baroreceptor sensitivity* contributes to orthostatic hypotension, causing dizziness on standing.
    - Decreased arterial compliance and vascular stiffness exacerbate BP-regulation difficulties.
    - Diuretic use may have led to dehydration, further aggravating his symptoms.

Management

- Gradual tapering of the diuretic dosage while maintaining fluid balance.
- Educate the patient on postural changes to minimize dizziness (e.g., rising slowly from a seated or lying position).
- Consider a different class of antihypertensive medication with less impact on blood pressure regulation.

Clinical Pearls

- Orthostatic hypotension is a common issue in the elderly due to reduced baroreceptor responsiveness.
- Medication regimens for hypertension must account for age-related cardiovascular changes and risks of falls.

Case 3: Nutritional Deficiencies and Gastrointestinal Function

Background

Ms K, a 74-year-old woman, complains of chronic fatigue, constipation, and frequent heartburn. She has a poor appetite and reports difficulty in swallowing certain foods. She takes a proton pump inhibitor (PPI) for GERD.

Discussion

Ms K's symptoms reflect GI changes associated with aging.

- *Key changes in GI system*:
    - Reduced *gastric acid secretion* impairs absorption of essential nutrients like calcium, iron, and vitamin B12.

- Weakened sphincter strength predisposes her to GERD symptoms.
- Slowed peristalsis contributes to her constipation.

Management

- Assess for nutrient deficiencies through serum tests (e.g., vitamin B12 and ferritin levels).
- Address constipation with increased dietary fiber, adequate hydration, and possible use of stool softeners.
- Consider reducing PPI dosage or switching to an H2-receptor antagonist to minimize nutrient malabsorption risks.

Clinical Pearls

- Chronic PPI use in the elderly can exacerbate nutrient deficiencies due to reduced gastric acid production.
- Management of constipation requires a multipronged approach, including dietary changes and physical activities.

These clinical scenarios emphasize the importance of understanding and addressing age-related physiological changes across systems. Effective management strategies include individualized treatment plans, close monitoring of medications, and lifestyle modifications tailored to the elderly patient's needs. By integrating these principles, healthcare providers can optimize care and improve outcomes for older adults.

CHANGES IN PHARMACOKINETICS IN THE ELDERLY

Pharmacokinetics refers to the processes of drug absorption, distribution, metabolism, and excretion. Age-related physiological changes alter these processes, which can impact the efficacy and safety of medications. This section explores these changes in detail with expanded examples and clinical implications.

Absorption

Absorption involves the movement of drugs from the site of administration into the bloodstream. In the elderly, the overall absorption rate of most drugs remains unchanged. However, specific physiological and pathological changes in the GI tract may influence certain drugs.

Key Changes in Absorption

- *Increased gastric pH*:
  - Age-related reduction in gastric acid secretion leads to a higher gastric pH (hypochlorhydria).
  - Drugs like calcium carbonate, iron salts, and ketoconazole, which require an acidic environment for absorption, show reduced bioavailability.
  - Conversely, drugs like aspirin that are stable in acidic environments may undergo altered absorption.
- *Slower gastric emptying and GI motility*:
  - Drugs such as paracetamol (acetaminophen) may have delayed onset of action due to slower gastric emptying.
  - This delay is exacerbated by conditions like diabetes gastroparesis, which are more common in the elderly.

- *Reduced first-pass metabolism:* Decreased hepatic extraction due to reduced liver perfusion increases the bioavailability of high first-pass drugs like propranolol, morphine, and verapamil, necessitating dose adjustments.
- *Topical and transdermal absorption*:
  - Aging skin becomes thinner with reduced blood flow, affecting the absorption of drugs from patches (e.g., fentanyl).
  - Elevated body temperature in febrile states can increase transdermal drug absorption, leading to potential toxicity.

Clinical Implications

- Drugs requiring active transport mechanisms, such as vitamin B12 and calcium, may have reduced absorption, leading to deficiencies.
- The increased bioavailability of certain drugs due to reduced first-pass metabolism necessitates careful dose adjustments to avoid toxicity.
- For drugs with delayed absorption, therapeutic monitoring may be needed to evaluate the timing and magnitude of the drug effect.

Table 8 outlines key physiological changes in drug absorption due to aging, providing examples of affected medications and their clinical consequences.

Distribution

Distribution refers to the movement of drugs from the bloodstream to tissues and organs. Age-related changes in body composition—such as increased fat, decreased water, and reduced lean body mass—can significantly alter drug distribution.

Key Changes in Distribution

- *Increased body fat:* Lipid-soluble drugs, such as diazepam, amiodarone, and propranolol, have a higher volume of distribution (Vd), leading to prolonged half-life and delayed drug elimination.
- *Decreased total body water:* Drugs that are water-soluble, such as aminoglycosides, digoxin, and ethanol, have a reduced Vd resulting in higher plasma concentrations and increased risk of toxicity.
- Reduced lean body mass: Medications such as digoxin, which is distributed to lean tissue, may accumulate at higher plasma levels increasing toxicity risk.
- *Serum protein binding:* Albumin, the primary binding protein for acidic drugs like warfarin and phenytoin, may decrease in malnourished or frail elderly patients, leading to increased free (active) drug levels.

TABLE 8: Age-related changes in drug absorption and their clinical implications.

Parameter	Age-related change	Examples	Clinical implications
Gastric pH	Increased	Calcium carbonate, iron, and ketoconazole	Reduced solubility of weakly acidic drugs
Gastric emptying	Slower	Paracetamol	Delayed onset of action
First-pass metabolism	Reduced hepatic extraction	Propranolol, morphine, and verapamil	Increased bioavailability

Alpha-1-acid glycoprotein, which binds basic drugs like propranolol and lidocaine, may increase during acute illness, temporarily altering drug binding dynamics.

Clinical Implications

- Lipophilic drugs accumulate in fat stores, increasing sedation and prolonging effects (e.g., benzodiazepines).
- Hydrophilic drugs show higher plasma concentrations, necessitating dose reductions to prevent toxicity.
- Close monitoring is required for protein-bound drugs to adjust for changes in free drug levels.

Table 9 highlights the effects of physiological changes in body composition and plasma protein levels on drug distribution in the elderly, illustrating examples and their clinical implications.

Metabolism

The liver is the primary site for drug metabolism, which involves converting drugs into active or inactive metabolites. Drug metabolism is classified into phase I (oxidation, reduction, and hydrolysis) and phase II (conjugation) reactions. Aging affects these pathways differently.

Key Changes in Metabolism:

- *Phase I metabolism*:
  - Phase I reactions mediated by cytochrome P450 enzymes (e.g., CYP1A2 and CYP2C19) decline with age, reducing the metabolism of drugs such as diazepam, theophylline, and amitriptyline.
  - CYP3A4 activity is variable and may remain unchanged or decline slightly.
- *Phase II metabolism:* Conjugation reactions (e.g., glucuronidation and sulfation) are generally preserved, making drugs like lorazepam and oxazepam safer options for elderly patients.
- *Hepatic blood flow*: Reduced hepatic blood flow decreases the clearance of drugs with high hepatic extraction ratios, such as propranolol, leading to prolonged drug half-lives.

Clinical Implications

- Drugs metabolized by phase I pathways (e.g., benzodiazepines) may require dose reductions due to prolonged clearance.

TABLE 9: Impact of age-related changes in drug distribution on pharmacokinetics.

Parameter	Age-related change	Examples	Clinical implications
Total body fat	Increased	Diazepam, amiodarone, and propranolol	Prolonged half-life of lipophilic drugs
Total body water	Decreased	Aminoglycosides, digoxin, and ethanol	Higher plasma concentrations
Serum albumin	Decreased	Warfarin and phenytoin	Increased free drug levels

TABLE 10: Age-related changes in hepatic metabolism and their clinical implications.

Parameter	Age-related change	Examples	Clinical implications
Phase I metabolism	Reduced CYP450 activity	Diazepam, theophylline, and amitriptyline	Prolonged clearance
Phase II metabolism	Unchanged	Lorazepam and oxazepam	Safer in elderly
Hepatic blood flow	Decreased	Propranolol	Prolonged half-life

- Drugs undergoing phase II metabolism are less affected by hepatic changes and are preferred in elderly patients.
- Frailty may further impair metabolic capacity, emphasizing the need for individualized drug dosing.

Table 10 summarizes how aging affects phase I and II metabolic pathways and hepatic blood flow, with examples of drugs impacted and their clinical consequences.

Excretion

Excretion is the removal of drugs from the body, primarily through the kidneys. Age-related decline in renal function is one of the most significant changes affecting pharmacokinetics in the elderly.

Key Changes in Renal Excretion

- *Decline in GFR:* GFR decreases by approximately 1% per year after the age of 40, leading to slower clearance of renally excreted drugs.
- *Reduced renal blood flow:* Renal perfusion declines by up to 50% by age 80, reducing the elimination of drugs like aminoglycosides and digoxin.
- *Tubular function:* Loss of tubular function impairs the reabsorption and secretion of drugs, increasing the risk of electrolyte imbalances and drug toxicity.
- *Serum creatinine misleading:* Reduced muscle mass leads to lower creatinine production, making serum creatinine levels appear "normal" even in the presence of significant renal impairment.

Clinical Implications

Renally excreted drugs (e.g., aminoglycosides, digoxin, and metformin) require dose adjustments based on estimated creatinine clearance (e.g., Cockcroft–Gault equation).

Monitoring renal function and serum drug levels is essential, especially for drugs with narrow therapeutic indices.

Table 11 outlines the effects of age-related renal function decline on drug clearance, highlighting examples of impacted drugs and the associated clinical risks.

Age-related changes in pharmacokinetics necessitate individualized drug selection, dose adjustments, and vigilant monitoring to optimize therapy and

TABLE 11: Age-related changes in renal excretion and their clinical implications

Parameter	Age-related change	Examples	Clinical implications
GFR	Declined by 25–50%	Digoxin, aminoglycosides, and metformin	Reduced clearance and drug accumulation
Renal blood flow	Decreased	NSAIDs	Increased risk of nephrotoxicity
Tubular function	Impaired	Diuretics	Risk of electrolyte imbalances

(GFR: glomerular filtration rate; NSAIDs: nonsteroidal anti-inflammatory drugs)

minimize adverse effects. By understanding the altered absorption, distribution, metabolism, and excretion of drugs in elderly patients, clinicians can ensure safer and more effective pharmacological management.

CLINICAL CASE SCENARIOS: PRACTICAL IMPLICATIONS OF AGE-RELATED CHANGES IN PHARMACOKINETICS

The following clinical case scenarios illustrate how age-related changes in PK (absorption, distribution, metabolism, and excretion) affect drug therapy in elderly patients. Each case demonstrates how these changes influence drug efficacy, safety, and clinical management.

Case 1: Absorption—Altered Gastric pH and First-pass Metabolism

Background

Mrs A, a 75-year-old woman, presents with fatigue and symptoms of anemia. She has a history of osteoporosis and has been taking calcium carbonate and iron supplements for several months without improvement in her symptoms. She also takes propranolol for hypertension.

Analysis

- *Absorption issues*:
  - *Increased gastric pH:* Mrs A's age-related hypochlorhydria (reduced gastric acid secretion) has likely reduced the absorption of calcium carbonate and iron, which require an acidic environment for optimal bioavailability.
  - *Reduced first-pass metabolism:* Propranolol, a high first-pass metabolism drug, may have increased bioavailability due to reduced liver perfusion, potentially resulting in lower BP and fatigue as side effects.

Management

- Switch from calcium carbonate to calcium citrate that is less dependent on gastric acid for absorption.
- Consider alternative formulations for iron supplementation, such as liquid preparations, or coadminister with vitamin C to enhance absorption.
- Monitor BP closely and reduce the propranolol dose if hypotension or fatigue persists.

Clinical Pearls

- Drugs like calcium carbonate and iron are less effective in elderly patients with reduced gastric acid secretion.
- Adjusting drug formulations or selecting alternatives can improve therapeutic outcomes in this population.

Case 2: Distribution—Increased Fat and Decreased Water

Background

Mr B, an 82-year-old man, presents to the emergency department with excessive drowsiness and confusion. His current medications include diazepam for anxiety and digoxin for heart failure. He has a history of heart failure and mild kidney dysfunction.

Analysis

- *Increased body fat:* Lipophilic drugs like diazepam are distributed into fat stores, increasing their Vd and prolonging their half-life. This can lead to drug accumulation and prolonged sedation.
- *Decreased total body water:* Water-soluble drugs like digoxin have a reduced Vd, resulting in higher plasma concentrations and increased risk of toxicity.

Management

- Discontinue diazepam and switch to a shorter-acting benzodiazepine, such as lorazepam, which is less affected by fat redistribution.
- Measure digoxin levels and adjust the dose to maintain therapeutic plasma concentrations.
- Educate the patient and caregiver about recognizing signs of drug toxicity, such as confusion, drowsiness, or arrhythmias.

Clinical Pearls

- Lipophilic drugs accumulate in fat stores, increasing the risk of prolonged effects in elderly patients.
- Water-soluble drugs have higher plasma concentrations, necessitating careful dose adjustments to avoid toxicity.

Case 3: Metabolism and Excretion—Impaired Hepatic and Renal Function

Background

Mrs C, an 85-year-old woman with a history of diabetes and atrial fibrillation, presents with nausea, decreased appetite, and confusion. Her medications include metformin for diabetes and warfarin for anticoagulation. Recent lab tests show mildly elevated serum creatinine and an international normalized ratio (INR) of 5.0.

Analysis

- *Impaired hepatic metabolism:* Warfarin, metabolized via CYP450 enzymes (phase I metabolism), has prolonged clearance due to reduced hepatic enzyme activity and blood flow. This has led to excessive anticoagulation, as indicated by an elevated INR.

- *Declined renal function:* Reduced GFR and tubular function impair the elimination of metformin, leading to drug accumulation and an increased risk of lactic acidosis, which may explain her nausea and decreased appetite.

Management

- Temporarily discontinue warfarin and monitor INR levels until they return to a safe range. Restart at a reduced dose with frequent monitoring.
- Hold metformin temporarily and assess renal function. If renal impairment persists, consider switching to alternative diabetes management, such as insulin.
- Monitor closely for signs of bleeding and acidosis. Educate the patient and caregivers about reporting symptoms like bruising, dark stools, or abdominal pain immediately.

Clinical Pearls

- Reduced phase I metabolism increases the half-life of drugs like warfarin, requiring close INR monitoring.
- Declined renal clearance necessitates dose adjustments or discontinuation of drugs like metformin to avoid toxic effects.

These case scenarios demonstrate the practical implications of age-related PK changes in elderly patients. Careful consideration of altered absorption, distribution, metabolism, and excretion is essential for optimizing drug therapy, preventing toxicity, and ensuring patient safety. Individualized treatment plans, regular monitoring, and patient education are key components of effective pharmacological management in older adults.

PHARMACODYNAMIC CHANGES IN THE ELDERLY

Pharmacodynamic changes in the elderly arise due to age-related alterations in receptor sensitivity, signal transduction pathways, and impaired homeostatic regulation. These changes significantly influence drug efficacy and the likelihood of ADEs.

Altered Receptor Sensitivity

β-adrenergic Receptors

- *Change:* Reduced density and diminished coupling to adenylate cyclase
- *Examples:*
    - β-blockers such as atenolol and propranolol demonstrate reduced effectiveness in elderly patients for controlling BP and heart rate.
    - Catecholamine-based drugs like isoproterenol show diminished responses due to these changes.
- *Clinical implications:* Alternative drugs, such as calcium channel blockers like amlodipine, are often preferred for managing hypertension and cardiovascular conditions.

Muscarinic Receptors

- *Change:* Decreased receptor density in the central nervous system (CNS).
- *Examples:* Increased sensitivity to anticholinergic drugs like diphenhydramine and tricyclic antidepressants (e.g., amitriptyline)
- *Clinical implications:* Avoidance of anticholinergic medications is critical due to risks of confusion, delirium, urinary retention, and constipation. The American Geriatrics Society (AGS) Beers Criteria strongly advises against the use of highly anticholinergic agents like amitriptyline and diphenhydramine.

Opioid Receptors

- *Change:* Reduced receptor density and endogenous opioid peptide levels
- *Examples:* Increased sensitivity to narcotics such as morphine and fentanyl, leading to a higher risk of respiratory depression and sedation
- *Clinical implications:* Initiate opioid therapy at lower doses and monitor closely for respiratory and CNS depression.

Alpha-1-adrenergic Receptors

- *Change:* Reduced receptor density in hepatic cells
- *Examples:* Drugs like midodrine, used for orthostatic hypotension, may show diminished efficacy.
- *Clinical implications:* Consider alternative therapeutic approaches for addressing metabolic and vascular issues.

Impaired Homeostatic Mechanisms

Baroreceptor Reflex

- *Change:* Blunted reflex sensitivity
- *Examples:* Medications like diuretics, nitrates, and α-blockers (e.g., prazosin) can cause significant orthostatic hypotension.
- *Clinical implications:* Educate patients to rise slowly from a seated or lying position to prevent falls. According to the AGS Beers Criteria, nonselective α-blockers are strongly discouraged in older adults.

Renin–angiotensin–aldosterone System

- *Change:* Reduced renin secretion and aldosterone production
- *Examples:* Angiotensin-converting enzyme (ACE) inhibitors (e.g., enalapril) and angiotensin receptor blockers (ARBs) (e.g., losartan) may lead to hyperkalemia due to altered potassium regulation.
- *Clinical implications:* Monitor potassium levels closely, especially when these drugs are combined with potassium-sparing diuretics or NSAIDs.

Thermoregulation

- *Change:* Diminished ability to maintain body temperature
- *Examples:* Anticholinergics can exacerbate hyperthermia by reducing sweat production, while sedatives increase hypothermia risk.
- *Clinical implications:* Avoid medications that disrupt temperature regulation in frail or immobile elderly patients.

Increased Sensitivity to Central Nervous System Drugs

Benzodiazepines

- *Change:* Heightened sensitivity to sedative and hypnotic effects.
- *Examples:* Medications like midazolam, lorazepam, and diazepam can cause excessive sedation, cognitive impairment, and increase the risk of falls.
- *Clinical implications:* Use short-acting benzodiazepines at the lowest effective dose. The Beers Criteria strongly advises against benzodiazepine use unless absolutely necessary.

Antipsychotics

- *Change:* Increased susceptibility to extrapyramidal symptoms (EPS) and tardive dyskinesia
- *Examples:* Haloperidol and risperidone can exacerbate these issues.
- *Clinical implications:* Use antipsychotics sparingly and monitor closely for movement disorders. Beers Criteria cautions against their use for behavioral problems in dementia unless nonpharmacologic options have failed.

Antidepressants

- *Change:* Increased risk of ADEs like hyponatremia and orthostatic hypotension
- *Examples:* Selective serotonin reuptake inhibitors (SSRIs) like sertraline can cause hyponatremia, while tricyclic antidepressants (e.g., amitriptyline) have anticholinergic effects.
- *Clinical implications:* Prefer SSRIs over tricyclics with regular electrolyte monitoring.

Specific Medications of Concern

Warfarin:

- *Change:* Enhanced anticoagulant effects due to reduced synthesis of clotting factors and plasma protein levels
- *Clinical implications:* Begin therapy at lower doses and monitor INR to avoid bleeding complications.

Digoxin:

- *Change:* Increased sensitivity to Na^+/K^+-ATPase inhibition.
- *Clinical implications:* Use lower doses in elderly patients, especially those with renal impairment. Avoid dosages >0.125 mg/day per Beers Criteria.

NSAIDs:

- *Change:* Increased GI and renal toxicity due to diminished mucosal defenses and renal perfusion
- *Clinical implications:* Use gastroprotective agents with NSAIDs or avoid long-term use entirely.

Table 12 synthesizes PD changes in the elderly with examples, clinical implications, and actionable recommendations to guide safe prescribing.

TABLE 12: Comprehensive overview of pharmacodynamic changes in the elderly.

Category	Change	Examples	Clinical implications	Recommendations
Receptor sensitivity				
β-adrenergic receptors	Reduced density and diminished coupling to adenylate cyclase	Atenolol, propranolol, and isoproterenol	Reduced effectiveness of β-blockers; diminished response to catecholamines	Use alternative drugs like calcium channel blockers (e.g., amlodipine) for cardiovascular conditions
Muscarinic receptors	Reduced density in CNS	Diphenhydramine and amitriptyline	Increased sensitivity to anticholinergics; higher risk of delirium, dry mouth, and constipation	Avoid anticholinergics; consider alternatives like SSRIs or loratadine for depression or allergies
Opioid receptors	Reduced receptor density	Morphine and fentanyl	Increased risk of sedation and respiratory depression	Start opioids at lower doses; monitor for toxicity
Alpha-1-adrenergic receptors	Reduced receptor density in hepatic cells	Midodrine	Impaired glycogenolysis; reduced effectiveness for orthostatic hypotension management	Consider alternative therapies; monitor glucose regulation
Homeostatic mechanisms				
Baroreceptor reflex	Blunted sensitivity to blood pressure changes	Diuretics, nitrates, and prazosin	Increased risk of orthostatic hypotension and falls	Educate patients to rise slowly; monitor for falls
RAAS	Reduced renin secretion and aldosterone production	ACE inhibitors (enalapril), ARBs (losartan)	Higher risk of hyperkalemia, especially with potassium-sparing diuretics or NSAIDs	Regularly monitor potassium and kidney function; avoid combining RAAS inhibitors with other risk drugs
Thermoregulation	Impaired ability to regulate body temperature	Anticholinergics and sedatives	Increased risk of hyperthermia or hypothermia	Avoid drugs that impair thermoregulation in frail elderly; monitor body temperature during extreme weather

Continued

Continued

Category	Change	Examples	Clinical implications	Recommendations
CNS sensitivity				
Benzodiazepines	Heightened sensitivity to sedative effects	Diazepam and lorazepam	Increased sedation, cognitive impairment, and risk of falls	Prefer short-acting agents at the lowest effective dose; avoid long-term use
Antipsychotics	Increased susceptibility to EPS and tardive dyskinesia	Haloperidol and risperidone	Higher risk of movement disorders and sedation	Use sparingly; prefer newer antipsychotics like quetiapine with careful monitoring
Antidepressants	Increased risk of hyponatremia and orthostatic hypotension	SSRIs (sertraline) and TCAs (amitriptyline)	Risk of falls, dizziness, and electrolyte imbalance	Monitor sodium levels; prefer SSRIs over TCAs for better safety
Specific drug classes				
Antihistamines	Strong anticholinergic effects	Diphenhydramine and promethazine	Delirium, urinary retention and dry mouth	Use safer alternatives like loratadine or cetirizine
NSAIDs	Increased GI bleeding and renal toxicity	Ibuprofen and naproxen	Risk of GI ulcers and kidney injury, especially with long-term use	Prescribe with PPIs for gastroprotection; limit use in high-risk patients
Warfarin	Enhanced anticoagulant effect	Warfarin	Increased bleeding risk due to reduced synthesis of clotting factors	Initiate therapy at a lower dose; closely monitor INR
Sulfonylureas	Increased risk of prolonged hypoglycemia	Glyburide and chlorpropamide	Higher risk of low blood glucose levels and adverse effects	Use short-acting agents like glipizide; avoid long-acting sulfonylureas.
Digoxin	Heightened sensitivity to Na^+/K^+-ATPase inhibition	Digoxin	Risk of toxicity, particularly in the presence of renal impairment	Dose adjustment based on renal function; monitor for nausea, visual changes, and arrhythmias
Anticoagulants	Enhanced bleeding risk due to intrinsic sensitivity	Warfarin	Increased sensitivity despite standard doses	Start at lower doses; maintain rigorous INR monitoring

(ACE: angiotensin-converting enzyme; ARB: angiotensin receptor blocker; CNS: central nervous system; EPS: extrapyramidal symptom; GI: gastrointestinal; INR: international normalized ratio; NSAID: nonsteroidal anti-inflammatory drugs; PPI: proton pump inhibitors; RAAS: renin–angiotensin–aldosterone system; SSRI: selective serotonin reuptake inhibitors; TCA: tricyclic antidepressant)

TABLE 13: Potentially inappropriate medications for the elderly.

Drug class/ medication	Example drugs	Recommendation	Rationale	Quality of evidence (QE)	Strength of recommendation (SR)
Antihistamines (first-generation)	Diphenhydramine, hydroxyzine, and meclizine	Avoid	Highly anticholinergic; increased risk of confusion, dry mouth, constipation, falls, and delirium	Moderate	Strong
Nitrofurantoin	Nitrofurantoin	Avoid in CrCl <30 mL/min or long-term use	Risk of pulmonary toxicity, hepatoxicity, and peripheral neuropathy	Low	Strong
Antipsychotics	Aripiprazole, haloperidol, and quetiapine	Avoid unless used for FDA-approved indications (e.g., schizophrenia and bipolar disorder)	Increased risk of stroke, cognitive decline, and mortality in dementia	Moderate	Strong
Benzodiazepines	Alprazolam, diazepam, and lorazepam	Avoid	Increased sensitivity; risk of cognitive impairment, delirium, falls, fractures, and motor vehicle crashes	Moderate	Strong
Nonbenzodiazepine hypnotics	Eszopiclone and zolpidem	Avoid	Similar risks to benzodiazepines, with minimal improvement in sleep latency or duration	Moderate	Strong
Tricyclic antidepressants (TCAs)	Amitriptyline, and nortriptyline	Avoid	Strong anticholinergic effects; risk of orthostatic hypotension and sedation	High	Strong
NSAIDs (nonselective)	Ibuprofen, naproxen, and diclofenac	Avoid chronic use unless gastroprotective agents are used	Increased risk of GI bleeding, peptic ulcer disease, kidney injury, and hypertension	Moderate	Strong
Warfarin	Warfarin	Avoid as initial therapy for atrial fibrillation or venous thromboembolism	Higher bleeding risk compared to DOACs; requires careful INR monitoring	High	Strong

Continued

Continued

Drug class/ medication	Example drugs	Recommendation	Rationale	Quality of evidence (QE)	Strength of recommendation (SR)
Skeletal muscle relaxants	Cyclobenzaprine and methocarbamol	Avoid	Poorly tolerated due to anticholinergic effects and sedation; increased risk of fractures	Moderate	Strong
Proton pump inhibitors (PPIs)	Omeprazole and pantoprazole	Avoid long-term use (>8 weeks) unless specific conditions warrant	Increased risk of *C. difficile* infections, pneumonia, and bone fractures	High	Strong
Insulin (sliding scale)	Short-acting insulin only	Avoid	Higher risk of hypoglycemia without significant improvement in blood glucose management	Moderate	Strong
Anticholinergics	Atropine and scopolamine	Avoid	Strong anticholinergic effects; increased risk of cognitive decline and falls	Moderate	Strong
Alpha-blockers (nonselective)	Doxazosin, and prazosin	Avoid for hypertension	High risk of orthostatic hypotension; safer alternatives available	Moderate	Strong
Opioids with benzodiazepines	Combination use	Avoid	Increased risk of sedation, respiratory depression, and overdose	Moderate	Strong
Sulfonylureas (long-acting)	Glyburide and glimepiride	Avoid	Increased risk of prolonged hypoglycemia compared to shorter-acting agents like glipizide	High	Strong
Dabigatran and rivaroxaban	DOACs	Avoid in severe renal impairment	Increased risk of bleeding in older adults with impaired renal function	Moderate	Strong

(CrCl: creatinine clearance; DOACs: direct oral anticoagulants: FDA: Food and Drug Administration; INR: international normalized ratio)

TABLE 14: Disease-specific drug recommendations.

Condition	Drugs to avoid	Reason
Delirium	Anticholinergics, benzodiazepines, and H2-receptor antagonists	Increased risk of cognitive decline and worsening delirium
Dementia/Cognitive impairment	Anticholinergics, antipsychotics, and benzodiazepines	Adverse CNS effects; increased risk of mortality in dementia
Falls/Fractures	Antidepressants (SSRIs and TCAs), antipsychotics, benzodiazepines	Increased risk of falls due to sedation and impaired psychomotor function
Parkinson disease	Metoclopramide, prochlorperazine, and promethazine	Dopamine-receptor antagonists exacerbate Parkinsonism
Heart failure	NSAIDs, COX-2 inhibitors, nondihydropyridine CCBs (e.g., diltiazem and verapamil)	Risk of fluid retention and worsening heart failure

(CCB: calcium channel blockers; CNS: central nervous system; NSAID: nonsteroidal anti-inflammatory drugs; SSRI: selective serotonin reuptake inhibitors; TCA: tricyclic antidepressant)

Integrating these insights into clinical practice helps mitigate risks and optimize therapeutic outcomes for elderly patients.

Table 13 is based on the detailed information extracted from the 2023 AGS Beers Criteria®. It summarizes medications and their respective recommendations, rationales, and potential risks for older adults, addressing various therapeutic classes and drug–disease interactions.

Table 14 represents the latest evidence-based guidelines for reducing inappropriate medication use and improving drug safety in elderly populations. Recommendations should be tailored to individual patients, considering their specific health conditions and therapeutic goals.

CLINICAL CASE SCENARIOS: PRACTICAL IMPLICATIONS OF AGE-RELATED PHARMACODYNAMIC CHANGES

Case Scenario 1: Managing Hypertension in the Elderly

Patient profile: A 78-year-old male with a history of hypertension and atrial fibrillation presents with poorly controlled BP. He is currently on atenolol and experiences fatigue and dizziness.

Pharmacodynamic changes impact:

- *β-adrenergic receptor alterations:* Reduced receptor density and coupling efficacy cause decreased responsiveness to atenolol.
- *Baroreceptor reflex blunting:* Impairs the body's ability to adjust BP postural changes, exacerbating dizziness.

Clinical Management

- Switch atenolol to a calcium channel blocker such as amlodipine, which acts independently of β-receptor sensitivity.

- Educate the patient on slow positional changes to mitigate orthostatic hypotension.
- Regularly monitor BP and renal function to assess drug efficacy and safety.

Outcome

Blood pressure is stabilized, and the patient reports improved energy levels and reduced dizziness.

Case Scenario 2: Addressing Pain Management in an Elderly Patient

Patient profile: An 82-year-old female with severe osteoarthritis is prescribed morphine for pain. After 1 week, she develops excessive sedation, confusion, and mild respiratory distress.

Pharmacodynamic changes impact:

- *Opioid receptor sensitivity:* Reduced receptor density but increased sensitivity to opioids leads to heightened risks of sedation and respiratory depression.
- *Impaired CNS homeostasis:* Decreased neurotransmitter levels exacerbate the sedative effects of opioids.

Clinical Management

- Reduce the morphine dose and consider transitioning to acetaminophen or a lower-potency opioid like tramadol.
- Monitor respiratory rate and signs of CNS depression closely.
- Address pain through adjunctive therapies, such as physical therapy or intra-articular injections, to minimize opioid dependence.

Outcome

The patient achieves adequate pain relief with no further sedation or respiratory issues.

Case Scenario 3: Preventing Adverse Effects of Polypharmacy

Patient profile: A 75-year-old male with diabetes, heart failure, and a recent history of a fall is taking metformin, lisinopril, and ibuprofen for chronic back pain. He presents with muscle weakness and fatigue.

Pharmacodynamic changes impact:

- *Renin-angiotensin-aldosterone system*: Reduced renin and aldosterone production increase the risk of hyperkalemia when using lisinopril.
- *NSAID-related toxicity:* NSAIDs exacerbate renal perfusion issues, contributing to fatigue and electrolyte imbalances.
- *Muscle weakness:* Likely due to mild hyperkalemia and reduced potassium excretion from the kidney.

Clinical Management

- Discontinue ibuprofen to reduce renal impairment risk and replace it with acetaminophen for pain management.

BOX 1 **Guidelines for rational prescribing in the elderly: Addressing age-related physiological and PK–PD changes.**

- *Nervous system*:
  - Avoid anticholinergic drugs: Medications such as diphenhydramine and amitriptyline should be avoided to reduce risks of confusion, delirium, and cognitive impairment
  - Limit use of benzodiazepines: Replace drugs like diazepam with short-acting alternatives such as lorazepam used sparingly due to risks of prolonged sedation and falls
  - Prescribe CNS drugs at lower doses: Initiate medications affecting the CNS, such as antidepressants, at reduced doses to minimize exaggerated sedative effects and toxicity
- *Cardiovascular system*:
  - Replace β-blockers when ineffective: Drugs like atenolol may have reduced efficacy due to decreased β-adrenergic receptor sensitivity. Consider calcium channel blockers like amlodipine for hypertension management
  - Monitor for orthostatic hypotension: Counsel patients on rising slowly from seated or lying positions when prescribing diuretics or α-blockers such as prazosin to prevent dizziness and fall risks
  - Limit nonspecific α-blockers: Avoid drugs like prazosin for hypertension, as they carry higher risks of postural hypotension in elderly patients
- *Respiratory system*:
  - Use caution with sedatives in COPD: Avoid sedatives like benzodiazepines or opioids for elderly patients with COPD to reduce the risk of respiratory depression
  - Avoid prolonged use of cough suppressants: Use codeine-based or similar suppressants cautiously to prevent mucus retention and an increased risk of respiratory infections
- *Gastrointestinal system*:
  - Limit long-term proton pump inhibitors (PPIs) use: Chronic use of PPIs such as omeprazole should be limited to <8 weeks when possible, to avoid risks of osteoporosis, hypomagnesemia, and nutrient malabsorption
  - Address nutritional deficiencies: Proactively prescribe vitamin B12, iron, or calcium supplements for elderly patients on long-term acid suppression therapy
  - Prefer stool softeners over laxatives: For constipation, avoid stimulant laxatives that may cause dependency. Use stool softeners, increased dietary fiber, and hydration as first-line options
- *Musculoskeletal system*:
  - Avoid nonessential corticosteroids: Limit corticosteroid use to prevent exacerbation of osteoporosis, sarcopenia, and fractures in elderly patients
  - Prescribe calcium and vitamin D: Supplement these nutrients to maintain bone health and reduce fracture risks in elderly individuals with osteoporosis or frailty
  - Encourage nonpharmacologic therapies for joint pain: Prioritize physical therapy and regular exercise over NSAIDs for managing osteoarthritis and joint stiffness
- *Endocrine system*:
  - Adjust antidiabetic medications: Use short-acting sulfonylureas like glipizide over long-acting agents such as glyburide to minimize risks of hypoglycemia in elderly diabetic patients
  - Monitor thyroid function regularly: Periodic testing of thyroid hormones is essential, as aging-related changes can necessitate dose adjustments for hypothyroidism or hyperthyroidism
- *Renal and urinary system*:
  - Adjust doses for renal clearance: Modify doses of renally excreted drugs like digoxin, metformin, and aminoglycosides based on estimated glomerular filtration rate (eGFR) to prevent accumulation and toxicity

Continued

Continued

- Avoid nephrotoxic drugs: Limit NSAIDs like ibuprofen and diclofenac in elderly patients with reduced renal function to minimize risks of acute kidney injury
- Promote bladder training: For elderly patients with urinary incontinence, emphasize nonpharmacologic approaches like bladder training and pelvic floor exercises before initiating medications like antimuscarinics

- *General recommendations*:
  - Educate about nonpharmacologic options: Integrate lifestyle modifications such as a balanced diet, regular physical activity, and physical therapy as first-line interventions before pharmacological treatments for chronic conditions

(CNS: central nervous system; COPD: chronic obstructive pulmonary disease; PD: pharmacodynamics; PK: pharmacokinetics; PPI: proton-pump inhibitor; NSAIDs: nonsteroidal anti-inflammatory drugs)

- Monitor potassium and renal function and adjust the lisinopril dose if needed.
- Educate the patient about nonpharmacologic approaches for managing back pain, such as physical therapy or heat therapy.

Outcome

The patient's potassium levels normalize, muscle weakness resolves, and there are no further falls.

Age-related PD changes underscore the need for tailored therapeutic strategies. By understanding receptor sensitivity changes, impaired homeostatic mechanisms, and CNS vulnerabilities, healthcare providers can mitigate adverse effects, improve outcomes, and ensure safer medication use for elderly patients.

Each case scenario highlights the importance of vigilant monitoring, appropriate drug substitutions, and patient education to optimize pharmacological management in the elderly.

Box 1 outlines tailored strategies for medication use in older adults, emphasizing the importance of minimizing adverse effects while ensuring therapeutic efficacy. The guidelines address changes in key physiological systems like the nervous, cardiovascular, respiratory, gastrointestinal, musculoskeletal, endocrine, and renal systems. Recommendations include avoiding anticholinergic drugs to prevent cognitive impairment, preferring nonpharmacologic interventions for joint pain and urinary incontinence, and using lower doses of CNS-acting drugs to mitigate sedation risks. Adjustments for renal clearance and proactive monitoring of thyroid and metabolic functions are highlighted to avoid drug accumulation and toxicity. **Box 1** underscores the need for replacing less effective or risky drugs with safer alternatives, such as calcium channel blockers over β-blockers or short-acting sulfonylureas over long-acting agents, and calls for educating patients about lifestyle modifications as first-line interventions to manage chronic conditions. These guidelines aim to optimize care and ensure safer medication practices for the elderly, particularly in the Indian context.

CONCLUSION

Aging profoundly affects the PD and PK of medications, underscoring the need for rational prescribing in the elderly. Through an understanding of age-related physiological changes—such as altered receptor sensitivity, impaired homeostatic mechanisms, and reduced renal and hepatic function—clinicians can enhance therapeutic outcomes and reduce ADEs.

Practical approaches, such as dose adjustments, careful drug selection, and regular monitoring, are critical to optimizing care in this vulnerable population. By integrating these principles into daily practice, healthcare providers can ensure safer, more effective treatments, ultimately improving the quality of life for elderly patients. The case scenarios presented illustrate the importance of individualized care and highlight strategies for addressing the complex interplay of aging and drug therapy.

This comprehensive understanding equips clinicians with the tools to navigate the challenges of prescribing for older adults, fostering patient-centered and evidence-based care.

SUGGESTED READINGS

1. Hämmerlein A, Derendorf H, Lowenthal DT. Pharmacokinetic and pharmacodynamic changes in the elderly. Clin Pharmacokinet. 1998;35(1):49-64.
2. Delafuente JC. Pharmacokinetic and pharmacodynamic alterations in the geriatric patient. Consult Pharm. 2008;23(4):324-34.
3. By the 2023 American Geriatrics Society Beers Criteria® Update Expert Panel. American Geriatrics Society 2023 updated AGS Beers Criteria® for potentially inappropriate medication use in older adults. J Am Geriatr Soc. 2023;71(7):2052-81.

3A

CHAPTER

Polypharmacy in the Elderly

ABSTRACT

Polypharmacy, defined as the concurrent use of five to nine medications, and hyperpolypharmacy, involving ten or more medications, are increasingly prevalent among older adults, particularly in India. Approximately 49% of older Indian adults experience polypharmacy, with 31% affected by hyperpolypharmacy, reflecting significant regional variations. While necessary for managing multimorbidity, polypharmacy heightens the risk of potentially inappropriate medications (PIMs), adverse drug events (ADEs), medication nonadherence, and other complications such as falls, cognitive impairment, and hospitalization. The issue is compounded by the prevalence of PIMs, which affects up to 28% of older adults in India, often due to a lack of regulation, generic prescribing, and suboptimal clinical guidelines.

Factors contributing to polypharmacy include an aging population, multimorbidity, fragmented healthcare systems, and unregulated prescribing practices. Strategies to mitigate polypharmacy emphasize clinical pharmacological reviews, judicious deprescribing, and adherence assessment. Tools such as the Beers criteria, Screening Tool of Older People's Prescriptions (STOPP)/the Screening Tool to Alert doctors to the Right Treatment (START) guidelines guidelines, and drug burden index aid in identifying high-risk medications. Deprescribing initiatives tailored to patient-specific care goals have demonstrated reductions in ADEs, hospitalizations, and healthcare costs.

A structured and individualized approach to medication management, involving informed reconciliation, therapeutic planning, and caregiver collaboration, is vital for optimizing elderly pharmacotherapy. The chapter underscores the importance of vigilance, clinical tools, and multidisciplinary involvement in addressing the challenges of polypharmacy to enhance patient outcomes and quality of life.

INTRODUCTION

Polypharmacy is defined as the concomitant use of five to nine medications, while hyperpolypharmacy is the use of ten or more medications.

The rising burden of chronic diseases among older adults necessitates complex medication regimens, leading to significant polypharmacy rates. A systematic review and meta-analysis revealed that approximately 49% of older Indian adults are affected by polypharmacy, while hyperpolypharmacy impacts 31% of this population. These figures underscore the widespread use of multiple medications among the elderly, raising concerns about the potential for inappropriate prescribing practices.

Regional variations exist, with Northeast India experiencing a polypharmacy prevalence of 65%, while hyper polypharmacy is notably higher in South India at 33%.

RISKS ASSOCIATED WITH POLYPHARMACY

The use of multiple medicines concomitantly increases the risk of the following issues:

- *Potentially inappropriate medications (PIMs)*: They are medications with high risk-benefit ratio for a particular individual or group of individuals
- *Adverse drug events (ADE)*: Potential drug-drug interactions (PDDIs) are defined as an increase or decrease in the therapeutic or adverse effect of a medication when given with another medication
- Medication nonadherence
- Increased healthcare costs
- Decreased functional status
- Increased cognitive impairment
- Increased falls
- Increased urinary incontinence
- Increased incidence of malnourishment
- Higher risk of hospitalization and death

Potentially inappropriate medications are particularly concerning about polypharmacy, with 28% of older adults in India reported to be on PIMs, which can lead to adverse drug reactions (ADRs) and diminished quality of life.

The use of PIMs is also unevenly distributed, with prevalence rates ranging from 17.8% in northern India to 33% in the west.

The adverse impacts of polypharmacy are further highlighted by its association with increased anticholinergic burden and cardiac autonomic neuropathy among community-dwelling elderly patients.

A study conducted in Kolkata, India, revealed that 26.6% were on polypharmacy. The study found that the anticholinergic burden, which refers to the cumulative effect of taking multiple medications with anticholinergic properties, was significantly higher among patients on polypharmacy and was associated with a higher incidence of cardiac autonomic neuropathy, a condition characterized by dysfunction in the autonomic nervous system, affecting cardiovascular health.

Moreover there are patients receiving medications that are not indicated, often due to prescribing by brand names instead of generic alternatives. This tendency increases healthcare costs and the risk of ADRs.

The literature reveals a high prevalence of ADRs, particularly among older adults with multiple comorbidities and those experiencing longer hospital stays.

Globally, it has been observed that up to half of the medications used by frail older patients are preventive in nature and often inappropriate or futile at the end of life. This scenario is similarly applicable in India, where there is a discrepancy between prescribed medications and the current health status and needs of elderly patients.

FACTORS CONTRIBUTING TO POLYPHARMACY IN ELDERLY PATIENTS

In India, the rapid aging of the population and the rising burden of chronic diseases have led to increased medication use, often resulting in polypharmacy and the use of PIMs. As people age, they develop more chronic conditions, known as multimorbidity. This creates difficulties for primary care physicians in the management of such patients, since clinical guidelines are typically limited to specific disease areas.

Patients may end up being prescribed multiple medications for each condition, leading to polypharmacy at an increased risk of adverse events and hospitalization.

This is compounded by a healthcare system dominated by the private sector, where 75% of healthcare expenses are out-of-pocket, causing significant financial strain on families.

The lack of regulation and standardization in prescribing practices exacerbates these issues, contributing to medication-related harm and ADRs.

STRATEGIES TO REDUCE POLYPHARMACY

Informed reconciliation for potential deprescribing need should be a norm in all patients receiving many medications for multiple chronic comorbidities.

Judicious deprescribing through clinical pharmacological review ensures better patient outcomes.

The review includes evaluation of the following:

- Drugs prescribed without indication
- Indication for a drug but none prescribed
- Too much or too little a dose
- Duplication of medications
- Drug-drug and drug-disease adverse interactions
- Nonadjustment of doses of medications as per comorbid diseases like renal impairment or hepatic disease
- ADRs and drug allergy
- Adherence issues
- Medication errors

The assessment of adherence, including methods patients use to manage medications, is of prime importance. The application of tools such as the *Morisky Medication Adherence scale* has validity in revealing breakdown in adherence and related barriers to taking medications.

The regimen in older persons is screened for high-risk drugs and those interacting with other drugs and affecting patient comorbidities. There is much information on high-risk drug therapy as defined by beers criteria, Screening Tool of Older People's Prescriptions (STOPP) guidelines, and drug burden index, and others. These tools help to identify therapy that has a high probability of ADEs compared with benefits in the older adult.

The trained clinical pharmacologist is equipped to assess the medications, indications, outcomes, and identify drug-therapy problems (DTPs) and propose a plan for optimizing therapy.

Recognition of DTPs within patients' medications is a crucial starting point for optimizing patients' medication regimens. Finally, the consultation should include an actionable therapeutic plan for optimizing medications within the patients' framework of their care goals. The plan is communicated with providers and is implemented and monitored with acceptance of the patient and caregiver.

Reducing polypharmacy by purposeful deprescribing has been shown to reduce medication-associated emergencies and hospitalizations, selectively. Deprescribing is best achieved within an individualized therapeutic plan that is understood by the patient and caregiver. It specifically targets high-risk drugs (inappropriate by criteria), overdosing, drug interactions and side effects, regimen simplification, improving adherence, and decreasing cost.

CONCLUSION

Polypharmacy is common and repeatedly shows associations with complications such as falls, hospitalizations, and mortality, regardless of which drugs are involved. The application of guidelines such as Beers and STOPP/START criteria recognize high-risk medications in older adults and are shown to avert ADEs and overall healthcare costs. Although useful, these do not fully capture entire nuances of clinical decision making for deprescribing in individual patients. Obtaining a comprehensive assessment and deprescribing plan is helpful in complex and transitional care situations. Careful vigilance for pharmacotherapy problems will always be important **(Box 1)**.

BOX 1 Recommendations for managing polypharmacy in the elderly.

- *Promote rational prescribing practices*:
  - Adhere to evidence-based guidelines, such as Beers criteria and STOPP/START recommendations, to identify and avoid high-risk medications
  - Use the drug burden index and other validated tools to assess and minimize anticholinergic and sedative loads
- *Implement structured medication reviews*:
  - Regularly evaluate medication regimens for appropriateness, necessity, and safety
  - Identify and address issues such as drug duplication, inappropriate indications, or contraindications
- *Focus on deprescribing*:
  - Develop individualized deprescribing plans for older adults with polypharmacy, targeting high-risk medications, and unnecessary preventive drugs
  - Engage patients and caregivers in deprescribing decisions to ensure adherence and acceptability

Continued

Continued

- *Enhance adherence monitoring*:
  - Assess adherence using validated tools like the Morisky Medication Adherence Scale
  - Address barriers to adherence, such as complex regimens, side effects, or financial constraints
- *Optimize doses based on patient characteristics*:
  - Adjust dosages for patients with renal or hepatic impairments
  - Tailor medications to the patient's comorbid conditions and overall health goals
- *Encourage multidisciplinary collaboration*:
  - Involve clinical pharmacologists, geriatricians, and primary care physicians in medication management
  - Foster communication between healthcare providers and caregivers to ensure continuity of care
- *Implement patient-centered therapeutic plans*:
  - Align medication regimens with the patient's care goals and quality-of-life considerations
  - Simplify regimens to reduce pill burden and enhance patient compliance
- *Educate patients and caregivers*:
  - Provide clear information on the purpose, benefits, and risks of each medication
  - Emphasize the importance of reporting side effects and maintaining regular follow-ups
- *Monitor for adverse drug events (ADEs)*:
  - Be vigilant for early signs of ADEs, particularly in high-risk populations
  - Establish protocols for managing ADEs promptly to prevent further complications
- *Strengthen regulatory and policy frameworks*:
  - Advocate for policies promoting generic prescribing and standardization of prescribing practices
  - Ensure accessibility of clinical decision-support systems for primary care providers

SUGGESTED READINGS

1. Nobili A, Marengoni A, Tettamanti M. Association between clusters of diseases and polypharmacy in hospitalized elderly patients: results from the REPOSI study. Eur J Intern Med. 2011;22(6):597-602.
2. Qato DM, Alexander GC, Conti RM. Use of prescription and over-the-counter medications and dietary supplements among older adults in the United States. JAMA. 2008;300(24):2867-78.
3. Leelakanok N, Holcombe AL, Lund BC. Association between polypharmacy and death: a systematic review and meta-analysis. J Am Pharm Assoc (2003). 2017;57(6):729-38.
4. Geitona M, Latsou D, Toska A. Polypharmacy and adherence among diabetic patients in Greece. Consult Pharm. 2018;33(10):562-71.
5. Maher RL, Hanlon J, Hajjar ER. Clinical consequences of polypharmacy in elderly. Expert Opin Drug Saf. 2014;13(1):57-65.
6. American Geriatrics Society 2015 Beers Criteria Update Expert Panel. American Geriatrics Society 2015 updated Beers criteria for potentially inappropriate medication use in older adults. J Am Geriatr Soc. 2015;63(11):2227-46.
7. Gallagher P, Ryan C, Byrne S. STOPP (Screening tool of older person's prescriptions) and START (screening tool to alert doctors to right treatment): consensus validation. Int J Clin Pharmacol Ther. 2008;46(2):72-83.
8. Salahudeen MS, Duffull SB, Nishtala PS. Anticholinergic burden quantified by anticholinergic risk scales and adverse outcomes in older people: a systematic review. BMC Geriatr. 2015;15:31.
9. Scott IA, Hilmer SN, Reeve E, Potter K, Le Couteur D, Rigby D, et al. Reducing inappropriate polypharmacy: the process of deprescribing. JAMA Intern Med. 2015;175(5):827-34.

3B
CHAPTER

Deprescribing: Concepts and Guidelines

ABSTRACT

Polypharmacy and inappropriate medication use are pervasive challenges in India's healthcare landscape, particularly among the elderly population. This chapter explores the concept of deprescribing as a critical intervention to mitigate the risks associated with polypharmacy, including adverse drug reactions (ADRs), medication nonadherence, and increased healthcare costs. It highlights the unique challenges within the Indian healthcare system, such as unregulated prescribing practices, antibiotic overuse, and limited reporting of adverse drug events (ADEs), emphasizing the need for deprescribing guidelines tailored to India's diverse healthcare settings.

The chapter outlines a structured framework for deprescribing, encompassing the identification of potentially inappropriate medications (PIMs) through tools such as the Beers Criteria and the Screening Tool of Older People's Prescriptions (STOPP)/the Screening Tool to Alert doctors to the Right Treatment (START) guidelines, CMRs, and shared decision-making strategies. It emphasizes a patient-centered approach, advocating for active patient and caregiver involvement in deprescribing decisions to align treatment plans with individual health goals and preferences.

Risk assessment methodologies, including the evaluation of drug–drug and drug–disease interactions, cumulative medication effects, and patient-specific factors, are detailed to optimize medication regimens and reduce adverse outcomes. The chapter also provides practical tapering and monitoring protocols to ensure safe medication discontinuation and long-term efficacy.

Implementation strategies focus on decision support tools, educational programs for healthcare providers, and policy advocacy to promote rational prescribing and deprescribing practices. Challenges such as cultural resistance, time constraints, and fear of negative outcomes are addressed with recommendations for system-wide improvements and workforce expansion.

By fostering a culture of "*no name, no shame, no blame*", the proposed deprescribing framework prioritizes collaboration, safety, and patient empowerment. The chapter underscores the transformative potential of deprescribing in India, aiming to improve patient safety, reduce healthcare costs, and enhance the overall quality of life for older adults. It concludes with recommendations for future research, integration of technology, and sustained advocacy to embed deprescribing practices into routine healthcare delivery.

INTRODUCTION

India's healthcare system faces numerous challenges related to medication management, exacerbating issues of polypharmacy, inappropriate prescribing, and medication misuse. The lack of regulation in the private sector results in significant variations in the quality and cost of services, contributing to inequitable access to healthcare.

While the public sector provides healthcare services at low or no cost, it is often perceived as unreliable and of inferior quality, which deters many individuals from seeking care unless they cannot afford private options. This perception and reality of varying quality levels complicate medication management, as the lack of consistent standards leads to a wide disparity in prescribing practices.

Another critical challenge is the overuse and misuse of medications, particularly antibiotics, in India. Studies have demonstrated that antibiotic overuse is prevalent across various regions, with pharmacists frequently dispensing antibiotics without prescriptions. This practice contributes to antibiotic resistance and poses a significant public health risk.

Polypharmacy is also widespread, with many patients receiving drugs without valid indications or due to prescribing by brand names instead of generic alternatives. This tendency increases healthcare costs and the risk of adverse drug reactions (ADRs). The literature reveals a high prevalence of ADRs, particularly among older adults with multiple comorbidities and those experiencing longer hospital stays. Contributing factors include poor prescribing practices and a lack of compliance with medication regimens.

Furthermore, there is a poor ADR reporting. Studies indicate that the low reporting rate is due to a lack of knowledge about the reporting process, time constraints, and fears of legal repercussions. This underreporting impedes efforts to identify and address medication-related problems effectively.

Addressing these challenges requires a multifaceted approach that includes regulatory reforms, increased government investment in healthcare, and initiatives to promote rational prescribing practices. Scaling up government expenditure on health could provide the necessary infrastructure boost, especially in rural and marginalized areas.

RATIONALE

The growing prevalence of polypharmacy and medication misuse among older adults in India highlights the urgent need for deprescribing guidelines tailored to the Indian healthcare context. In India, the rapid aging of the population and the rising burden of chronic diseases have led to increased medication use, often resulting in polypharmacy and the use of potentially inappropriate medications (PIMs).

Structured guides to deprescribing, which include algorithms and flowcharts, can aid clinicians in systematically reviewing and discontinuing medications that are no longer necessary or potentially harmful. In the Indian context, this opinion would provide a framework for healthcare providers to evaluate and optimize medication regimens, ensuring they align with the patient's current health needs and circumstances.

The healthcare providers need to critically evaluate prescribing practices without fear of retribution or embarrassment. By focusing on improving patient outcomes rather than assigning blame, guidelines should promote a culture of safety and continuous improvement in medication management.

The principle of no name, no shame, no blame supports collaborative decision-making, allowing healthcare providers to work together with patients and caregivers to tailor medication regimens that are both effective and appropriate for the individual's current health status and goals. By fostering a system where learning and adaptation are prioritized, these guidelines aim to significantly enhance the quality of care for older adults in India, ultimately leading to better health outcomes and reduced healthcare costs.

The following are the steps of progression in the deprescribing journey.

Identifying Potentially Inappropriate Medications

Identifying PIMs is a crucial first step in the deprescribing process. PIMs are medications where the potential risks outweigh the benefits, particularly in older adults who are more susceptible to ADRs due to age-related changes in pharmacokinetics and pharmacodynamics. The identification of PIMs involves using standardized screening tools and conducting comprehensive medication reviews (CMRs) to optimize medication regimens and improve patient outcomes.

Use of Screening Tools

Beers Criteria

The Beers Criteria, developed by the American Geriatrics Society, is one of the most widely used tools for identifying PIMs in older adults. It provides a list of medications that are potentially inappropriate for use in older populations, based on their association with an increased risk of adverse effects.

Key features: The Beers Criteria categorizes medications into different lists based on the type of risk they pose, such as medications to avoid regardless of condition, medications to avoid in certain diseases or syndromes, and medications to use with caution. It also provides recommendations for alternative therapies when available.

Application in practice: Healthcare providers can use the Beers Criteria as a reference during medication reviews to identify medications that may no longer be appropriate for older adults. For example, medications with strong anticholinergic properties, such as diphenhydramine, are included in the list due to their potential to cause confusion, dry mouth, constipation, and urinary retention in elderly patients.

STOPP/START Criteria

The Screening Tool of Older People's Prescriptions (STOPP) and the Screening Tool to Alert doctors to the Right Treatment (START) provide a complementary approach to identify PIMs and prescribing omissions.

STOPP criteria: This tool helps identify medications that are potentially inappropriate based on physiological changes in older adults and the risk of drug-drug and drug-disease interactions. For instance, the use of long-term benzodiazepines for anxiety in elderly patients is discouraged due to the risk of sedation and falls.

START criteria: In contrast, the START criteria focus on identifying therapeutic gaps where patients are not receiving medications that are clinically indicated for their conditions. For example, it alerts healthcare providers to consider statins for older adults with a history of coronary artery disease unless contraindicated.

Clinical use: The STOPP/START criteria can be used in conjunction with the Beers Criteria to provide a more comprehensive assessment of medication appropriateness. This approach ensures that clinicians not only identify PIMs but also address under-treatment by ensuring that necessary medications are not omitted.

Comprehensive Medication Review Process

A CMR is an in-depth evaluation of a patient's medication regimen with the goal of identifying PIMs, optimizing therapy, and improving patient outcomes. This process involves several key steps.

Medication Reconciliation

Objective: Ensure that the medication list is accurate and complete by verifying the medications, doses, and frequencies with the patient and cross-referencing with their medical records.

Process: Engage patients in reviewing their medication lists, including prescription drugs, over-the-counter medications, supplements, and herbal products. Identify any discrepancies, such as duplicate therapies or omissions, and reconcile them with the healthcare team.

Assessment of Medication Indications and Effectiveness

Objective: Evaluate each medication for its current indication and therapeutic effectiveness. Determine if the medication is still necessary and if it achieves the desired outcomes.

Considerations: Assess whether the patient's condition or therapeutic goals have changed and whether there are more effective or safer alternatives. For example, long-term proton pump inhibitor use should be reassessed for patients who no longer have indications such as peptic ulcer disease or chronic gastroesophageal reflux disease.

Evaluation of Adverse Effects and Drug Interactions

Objective: Identify any adverse effects or drug-drug interactions that may be harmful or contribute to new symptoms. This includes assessing the cumulative effect of medications with similar side effect profiles.

Tools: Utilize tools like the Anticholinergic Burden Scale to evaluate the cumulative anticholinergic effect, which can impair cognitive function and increase fall risk in older adults.

Assessment of Adherence and Patient Preferences

Objective: Evaluate patient adherence to the medication regimen and understand any barriers they may face, such as complexity of the regimen, cost, or side effects.

Approach: Engage patients in discussions about their medication experiences and preferences. This includes understanding their goals and aligning the medication plan with their values and lifestyle.

Documentation and Follow-up

Objective: Document the findings of the medication review, including any changes made to the regimen, the rationale for those changes, and the anticipated outcomes.

Plan: Establish a follow-up plan to monitor the effects of any changes and address any new concerns that may arise. Regular follow-ups help ensure the medication regimen remains optimal over time.

In conclusion, the identification of PIMs is a foundational step in the deprescribing process, critical for enhancing patient safety and optimizing therapeutic outcomes, particularly among the elderly in India.

The application of screening tools such as the Beers Criteria and STOPP/START Criteria offers healthcare providers a robust framework for evaluating medication appropriateness. These tools facilitate the identification of both PIMs and undertreatment, ensuring that medication regimens are tailored to the unique needs of each patient.

The CMR process proposed as clinical pharmacological reconciliation, review, and feedback (CPRRF) further supports this effort by enabling a detailed assessment of medication indications, effectiveness, and potential adverse effects, while actively engaging patients in discussions about their treatment preferences and adherence challenges.

Their involvement is particularly crucial for the elderly population at risk of polypharmacy and associated complications such as anticholinergic burden and cardiac autonomic neuropathy.

Risk Assessment

Effective risk assessment in deprescribing involves evaluating drug-drug interactions, drug-disease interactions, and considering cumulative effects alongside patient-specific factors. This comprehensive approach helps in minimizing potential adverse outcomes and optimizing therapeutic efficacy, particularly in older adults who often have complex medication regimens.

Evaluation of Drug–drug and Drug–disease Interactions

Drug-drug interactions occur when the pharmacological effects of one medication are altered by the presence of another. Drug-disease interactions happen when a medication exacerbates a patient's existing medical condition. Both types of interactions can lead to increased morbidity, especially in older adults who are more likely to be on multiple medications for various comorbidities.

Methods for Evaluation

- *Medication review*: Regular CMRs are crucial. These involve assessing the entire medication regimen to identify potential interactions and adjust prescriptions accordingly. This review should incorporate patient history, existing health conditions, and all current medications, including over-the-counter drugs and supplements.
- *Clinical decision support systems (CDSS)*: Utilizing technology to support decision-making in prescribing practices can alert healthcare providers to potential interactions at the point of care.
- *Consultation with clinical pharmacologists*: Involving clinical pharmacologist (DM clinical pharmacology) or in absence of clinical pharmacologist, pharmacologist with basic medical degree in the healthcare team can provide additional expertise in identifying and managing drug–drug and drug–disease interactions. They can offer insights into alternative therapies and assist in optimizing medication regimens.

Consideration of Cumulative Effects and Patient-specific Factors

Cumulative effects refer to the overall impact of multiple medications on a patient's health, considering pharmacokinetics and pharmacodynamics. Patient-specific factors include age, weight, kidney and liver function, genetic factors, and individual health goals.

Cumulative Effects

- *Anticholinergic burden*: A high anticholinergic burden can lead to cognitive impairment, confusion, and increased risk of falls, particularly in older adults. Tools such as the Anticholinergic Burden Scale can help evaluate the cumulative anticholinergic effect of a patient's medication regimen.
- *Sedative load*: Similar to the anticholinergic burden, the cumulative sedative load should be assessed to prevent excessive sedation, which can impair mobility and cognitive function. This assessment is particularly relevant in patients on multiple medications with sedative properties.

Patient-specific Factors

- *Comorbidities*: The presence of multiple chronic diseases can affect how medications interact with each other and with the body. Risk assessment should consider how each medication aligns with the patient's overall health profile.
- *Functional*: Evaluating the patient's functional status, including cognitive and physical capabilities, is crucial. Medications should be aligned with the patient's ability to manage their regimen and with their lifestyle. For instance, consider an elderly patient who is prescribed multiple medications for comorbidities and needs to take several pills at different times of the day. The patient finds it challenging to remember the timing and often misses doses, leading to poor control of targets.

  To align the medication plan with the patient's ability to manage it, the prescribing physician could:

   - Consolidate dosing times: Adjust the schedule so that medications are taken at the same time each day, such as morning and evening, to reduce confusion.
   - Use combination medications: Where possible, switch to combination pills (e.g., a single pill containing both a blood pressure medication and a statin) to decrease the number of pills the patient needs to take.
   - Switch to once-daily formulations: Replace medications that require multiple daily doses with once-daily alternatives, if available and effective, to simplify the regimen.
   - Use medication aids: Recommend using a pill organizer or setting up reminders on a mobile device to help the patient remember to take their medications.
- *Patient preferences and goals*: Engaging patients in shared decision-making ensures that their preferences and health goals are considered. This collaborative approach helps align treatment plans with what patients' value most in their care. While concerns about engaging patients in shared decision-making in India may arise due to illiteracy rates, this barrier can be effectively addressed through culturally sensitive communication strategies and patient-centered approaches. Illiteracy does not equate to a lack of understanding or inability to participate in healthcare decisions.

By *using simple language*, visual aids, and local dialects, healthcare providers can convey complex medical information in a way that is accessible and comprehensible.

Additionally, *involving family members*, who often play a crucial role in healthcare decisions in India, can help bridge gaps in understanding. By actively listening to the patient's concerns and values, even those with limited formal education can express their preferences and priorities. This collaborative approach ensures that treatment plans are aligned with what patients' value most in their care, leading to better adherence and outcomes. The success of shared decision-making in such contexts lies in the healthcare provider's ability to adapt their communication style and engage the patient and family members meaningfully in the care process.

Strategies for Risk Assessment

- *Risk scoring systems*: Implementing risk scores, such as the GerontoNet ADR risk score, helps estimate the likelihood of ADRs based on patient-specific factors such as age, comorbidities, and renal function.
- *Regular monitoring and follow-up*: Continuous monitoring of the patient's response to medication changes and regular follow-ups are essential to adapt treatment plans as needed and to prevent adverse events.

A thorough risk assessment process that incorporates evaluations of drug-drug and drug-disease interactions, as well as patient-specific factors and cumulative effects, is essential for optimizing medication regimens. By using a patient-centered approach and leveraging available tools and resources, healthcare providers can enhance patient safety and improve therapeutic outcomes in older adults.

Patient-centered Approach

Strategies for Shared Decision-making

Shared decision-making is a collaborative process that involves healthcare providers and patients working together to make decisions about the patient's care. In the context of deprescribing, this approach is critical to ensuring that patients' preferences, values, and needs are considered, leading to more personalized and acceptable medication plans.

Engagement and Communication

Patient involvement: Encouraging patients to actively participate in their healthcare decisions fosters a sense of ownership and empowerment. Clinicians should facilitate open discussions about the risks and benefits of medications, emphasizing that the goal is to optimize health outcomes and minimize harm.

Building trust: Establishing a trusting relationship between patients and healthcare providers is essential for effective shared decision-making. This involves listening to patients' concerns, respecting their autonomy, and providing information transparently and empathetically.

Information Sharing

Education on medication effects: Patients should be informed about how medications affect their bodies, especially as they age, which may necessitate changes in medication regimens. Discussions should include potential side effects, interactions, and the possibility of ADRs.

Exploration of alternatives: Presenting alternative treatment options, including nonpharmacological approaches, allows patients to consider various pathways to managing their health conditions. This can include lifestyle changes, dietary modifications, or the use of supplements.

Decision Aids

Utilization of decision aids: Tools such as decision aids can help patients understand their options and the potential outcomes of continuing, reducing, or stopping medications. These aids can be brochures, charts, or digital applications that visually represent information.

Collaborative goal setting: Working with patients to set realistic and achievable health goals is an integral part of the decision-making process. This ensures that the deprescribing plan aligns with the patient's life goals and expectations.

Individualized Care Planning

Individualized care planning tailors medical interventions to the unique needs and circumstances of each patient. This approach recognizes that each patient's health journey is different and requires personalized strategies to achieve optimal outcomes

Comprehensive Assessment

Holistic evaluation: Assessing a patient's overall health status, including their physical, mental, and social well-being, provides a complete picture necessary for personalized care planning. This includes understanding the patient's lifestyle, social support systems, and health literacy.

Risk-benefit analysis: Evaluating the potential risks and benefits of each medication in the context of the patient's current health status is crucial. Factors such as comorbidities, life expectancy, and functional abilities should guide the deprescribing process.

Tailored Interventions

Customized medication plans: Adjusting medication regimens based on individual patient factors, such as genetics, preferences, and responses to treatment, ensures that each patient receives the most appropriate care. This includes dose adjustments, substitution with safer alternatives, or discontinuation.

Monitoring and follow-up: Regular monitoring of patient outcomes and ongoing communication are essential components of individualized care. This allows for timely adjustments to the care plan and addresses any emerging issues, such as withdrawal symptoms or the recurrence of symptoms.

Patient and Caregiver Involvement

Collaborative care models: Involving caregivers and family members in the care process can enhance support and adherence to deprescribing plans. Their insights and observations can provide valuable information about the patient's response to medication changes.

Empowerment and education: Empowering patients and caregivers with knowledge about medication management promotes adherence and proactive health management. Educational initiatives should focus on recognizing ADRs, understanding medication labels, and the importance of adherence.

A patient-centered approach to deprescribing emphasizes the importance of shared decision-making and individualized care planning. By actively involving patients in their healthcare decisions and tailoring interventions to their specific needs, healthcare providers can improve patient outcomes, enhance satisfaction, and ensure the safe and effective use of medications. This approach aligns with the broader goals of deprescribing to minimize medication burden and optimize therapeutic benefits.

Prioritization Framework for Deprescribing

Criteria for Prioritizing Medications for Deprescription

The process of deprescribing involves the careful evaluation of a patient's medication regimen to identify PIMs and prioritize those that should be discontinued or adjusted. The prioritization framework for deprescribing is essential to optimize patient safety and enhance therapeutic outcomes. The following criteria are crucial in determining which medications should be prioritized for deprescription:

- *Potential for harm*: Medications that pose a high risk of adverse effects, particularly in vulnerable populations such as the elderly, should be prioritized for review. This includes drugs with a high anticholinergic burden, sedative properties, or those that increase the risk of falls, cognitive impairment, or cardiovascular events.

- *Lack of indication*: Medications that are not supported by a clear clinical indication or whose therapeutic goals have been achieved should be considered for discontinuation. This includes medications prescribed for conditions that are no longer present or for symptoms that have resolved.
- *Redundancy*: Medications with overlapping mechanisms of action or therapeutic effects should be assessed for redundancy. This often occurs when multiple medications are prescribed for the same condition, and leading to unnecessary polypharmacy.
- *Patient preference and quality of life*: Patient-centered care involves considering the patient's preferences and quality of life when making deprescribing decisions. Medications that adversely affect a patient's quality of life or do not align with their treatment goals should be prioritized for discontinuation.
- *Drug-drug and drug-disease interactions*: Medications that have significant interactions with other drugs or exacerbate existing medical conditions should be reviewed. This includes drugs that may worsen comorbid conditions or interact negatively with other therapies.
- *Pharmacoeconomic considerations*: The cost of medications should be considered, especially for elderly patients who may have limited financial resources. When a less expensive but equally effective alternative is available, it should be prioritized to reduce the economic burden. Deprescribing or switching to cost-effective options can help manage healthcare expenses, making treatments more accessible and sustainable for patients who live frugally due to limited savings or cash flow. This approach aligns with patient-centered care by considering the financial impact of medication regimens on the patient's overall quality of life.

PROCESS FOR PRIORITIZATION BASED ON RISK AND BENEFIT ANALYSIS

The prioritization process for deprescribing involves a systematic assessment of the risks and benefits associated with each medication. The following steps outline the process for prioritization:

- *Medication reconciliation*: Conduct a comprehensive review of the patient's current medication list, including prescription drugs, over-the-counter medications, and supplements. This step ensures that all medications are accounted for and provides a basis for further evaluation.
- *Risk assessment*: Evaluate the risk associated with each medication, considering factors such as the patient's age, renal and hepatic function, and comorbidities. Tools such as the Anticholinergic Burden Calculator and risk scales can aid in assessing the cumulative risk associated with multiple medications.
- *Benefit analysis*: Assess the therapeutic benefits of each medication in the context of the patient's current health status and treatment goals. Consider

whether the medication achieves its intended outcomes and whether alternative therapies might offer a better risk-benefit profile.

- *Clinical judgment and shared decision-making*: Engage the patient and their caregivers in the decision-making process. Discuss the risks and benefits of continuing or discontinuing each medication, considering the patient's preferences and values.
- *Implementation and monitoring*: Once a decision is made to discontinue or adjust a medication, implement a tapering plan if necessary and monitor the patient for withdrawal symptoms or changes in their condition. Regular follow-ups are essential to ensure the safety and efficacy of the deprescribing process.
- *Documentation*: Document the rationale for deprescribing decisions, including the anticipated outcomes and any discussions with the patient. This documentation is vital for continuity of care and for communicating with other healthcare providers involved in the patient's care.

By employing a structured prioritization framework, healthcare providers can effectively manage polypharmacy and reduce the risk of adverse drug events. This approach not only enhances patient safety but also improves the overall quality of care by ensuring that medication regimens are aligned with the patient's current health needs and treatment goals.

TAPERING AND MONITORING PROTOCOLS

Effective deprescribing requires careful planning and monitoring to ensure patient safety and improve outcomes. This section provides guidelines for the safe tapering of medications and outlines strategies for monitoring and follow-up during the deprescribing process.

Process of Safe Tapering of Medications

Assess the Need for Tapering

Before initiating tapering, evaluate whether tapering is necessary based on the patient's current health status, risk of withdrawal symptoms, and overall treatment goals. Consider the pharmacokinetics and pharmacodynamics of the medication, particularly for those with a long half-life or those that are highly potent.

Medications that commonly require tapering include benzodiazepines, antidepressants, antipsychotics, and corticosteroids due to the risk of withdrawal symptoms or rebound effects.

Develop a Tapering Schedule

Create a tapering schedule tailored to the individual patient, considering factors such as the dosage, duration of use, and patient's response to previous tapering attempts.

Start with a small reduction in dose, typically 10–25% of the current dose, and adjust based on patient tolerance and response.

Allow sufficient time between dose reductions to monitor for withdrawal symptoms and to allow the patient to adjust physiologically and psychologically.

Monitor for Withdrawal Symptoms

Educate patients and caregivers about potential withdrawal symptoms and encourage them to report any adverse effects promptly.

Common withdrawal symptoms may include anxiety, insomnia, agitation, and physical symptoms such as nausea or dizziness.

Adjust the tapering schedule if significant withdrawal symptoms occur, possibly slowing the rate of tapering or pausing to stabilize the patient.

Patient Education and Support

Engage patients in shared decision-making, ensuring they understand the reasons for tapering and are involved in the planning process.

Provide educational resources and support throughout the tapering process to improve adherence and confidence.

Monitoring Strategies and Follow-up Plans

Regular Monitoring Visits

Schedule regular follow-up visits to assess the patient's response to tapering, monitor for withdrawal symptoms, and make necessary adjustments to the tapering plan.

Use these visits to reassess the patient's overall medication regimen and address any new or ongoing health concerns.

Use of Monitoring Tools

Implement tools such as the Anticholinergic Burden Calculator or medication review checklists to identify potential risks and assess the effectiveness of the deprescribing process.

Consider using clinical informatics tools like the Geriatric Risk Assessment MedGuide (GRAM) for identifying and managing risks associated with polypharmacy.

Interdisciplinary Collaboration

Collaborate with pharmacists, nurses, and other healthcare providers to ensure comprehensive care and support during the tapering process.

Engage in discussions with specialists when managing complex cases or when new medications are introduced.

Patient Feedback and Adjustment

Encourage patients to provide feedback about their experiences and any difficulties encountered during tapering.

Be prepared to adjust the tapering strategy based on patient feedback and clinical findings.

Long-term Follow-up

After completing the tapering process, continue to monitor the patient's health status, and medication regimen periodically to prevent the reintroduction of unnecessary medications.

Focus on maintaining an optimal medication regimen that aligns with the patient's current health needs and goals.

The process of tapering and monitoring medications during deprescribing is a patient-centered approach that requires careful planning, interdisciplinary collaboration, and ongoing evaluation to achieve safe and effective outcomes. Implementing these strategies will help mitigate the risks associated with polypharmacy and improve the quality of care for older adults.

Implementation Strategies

Implementing deprescribing guidelines effectively requires a comprehensive approach involving appropriate tools, educational programs, and strategies to overcome challenges and barriers. This section outlines the tools and resources developed to support guideline implementation, describes educational programs for healthcare providers, and discusses the challenges faced during implementation along with potential strategies to address them.

Tools and Resources

A variety of tools and resources have been developed to facilitate the implementation of deprescribing guidelines. These include decision support algorithms, educational pamphlets, and web-based resources designed to assist healthcare providers and patients in the deprescribing process.

Decision Support Algorithms

Decision support algorithms are central to the implementation of deprescribing guidelines. These algorithms provide healthcare providers with a step-by-step framework for evaluating and discontinuing PIMs. By integrating these algorithms into electronic health records (EHRs), clinicians can easily access them during patient consultations, ensuring that deprescribing considerations are part of routine care.

Educational Pamphlets and Web-based Resources

Educational pamphlets and web-based resources have been developed to inform patients about the benefits and processes of deprescribing. These materials aim to increase patient engagement and understanding, empowering them to participate actively in decision-making about their medications. Web-based resources also offer interactive tools, such as medication review checklists and risk assessment calculators, to assist both patients and healthcare providers in identifying medications suitable for deprescribing.

Integration with Clinical Practice Guidelines

Incorporating deprescribing recommendations within existing clinical practice guidelines is crucial for widespread adoption. By embedding these recommendations into standard care protocols, healthcare providers are more likely to consider deprescribing as part of their regular practice. Collaboration with guideline development organizations can facilitate this integration, ensuring that deprescribing is included in the treatment pathways for various conditions.

Educational Programs

Education and training programs are essential components of implementing deprescribing guidelines. These programs are designed to equip healthcare providers with the knowledge and skills needed to effectively carry out deprescribing in clinical practice.

Training Workshops and Seminars

Training workshops and seminars offer healthcare providers the opportunity to learn about the principles and practices of deprescribing. These sessions typically cover topics such as identifying PIMs, conducting CMRs, and engaging in shared decision-making with patients. By providing hands-on training and real-world scenarios, these programs enhance clinicians' confidence and competence in deprescribing.

Interprofessional Education

Interprofessional education (IPE) programs bring together healthcare providers from different disciplines to learn about deprescribing collaboratively. These programs emphasize the importance of teamwork and communication in the deprescribing process, highlighting the roles of various healthcare professionals, including physicians, pharmacists, nurses, and social workers, in optimizing medication use.

Online Learning Modules

Online learning modules offer flexible and accessible training options for healthcare providers. These modules provide comprehensive coverage of deprescribing concepts and practices, allowing clinicians to learn at their own pace. Interactive elements, such as quizzes and case studies, reinforce learning, and provide opportunities for self-assessment.

Challenges and Barriers

Despite the availability of tools and educational programs, several challenges and barriers can hinder the implementation of deprescribing guidelines. Understanding these obstacles is critical to developing strategies to overcome them.

Cultural and Organizational Barriers

One of the primary challenges in implementing deprescribing guidelines is the existing culture within healthcare organizations that prioritizes prescribing over deprescribing. Many healthcare providers are accustomed to prescribing medications and may be resistant to discontinuing them, fearing potential negative outcomes, or perceived challenges to their clinical judgment.

Lack of Time and Resources

Healthcare providers often face time constraints during patient consultations, making it difficult to conduct thorough medication reviews and engage in detailed discussions about deprescribing. Additionally, limited access to resources, such as clinical pharmacologists or decision support tools, can further impede the implementation process.

Fear of Negative Outcomes

Concerns about negative outcomes, such as withdrawal symptoms or the recurrence of medical conditions, can deter healthcare providers from deprescribing. This fear is compounded by a lack of robust evidence and clear guidelines on managing such outcomes, leading to hesitation in initiating deprescribing interventions.

Discussion

The discussion section of this opinion provides an overview of their anticipated impact on patient outcomes, a comparison with existing international deprescribing guidelines, and suggestions for future research and refinement.

IMPACT ON PATIENT OUTCOMES

Implementing these deprescribing opinions is expected to significantly enhance patient safety and quality of life by optimizing medication regimens and reducing the risks associated with polypharmacy. The guidelines aim to achieve the following benefits:

- *Reduction in adverse drug events*: By identifying and discontinuing PIMs, the guidelines aim to decrease the incidence of adverse drug events, which are particularly prevalent among older adults due to the complex nature of their medication regimens. Studies have shown that reducing polypharmacy can lower the risk of hospitalizations and emergency department visits.
- *Improvement in cognitive and physical function*: Deprescribing medications that contribute to anticholinergic burden or have sedative properties can lead to improvements in cognitive and physical function, thereby enhancing the overall quality of life for older adults.
- *Increased patient engagement and satisfaction*: By emphasizing patient-centered care and shared decision-making, the guidelines foster greater patient involvement in their healthcare. Engaged patients are more likely to adhere to treatment plans, experience improved outcomes, and report higher levels of satisfaction with their care.
- *Optimized medication use*: The guidelines encourage healthcare providers to regularly assess the appropriateness of medications, leading to more rational and targeted use of pharmacotherapy. This optimization can result in cost savings for both patients and healthcare systems by reducing unnecessary medication use and associated costs.

COMPARISON WITH INTERNATIONAL GUIDELINES

These guidelines align with international deprescribing guidelines while also addressing specific considerations relevant to the Indian healthcare context:

- *Beers Criteria and STOPP/START Criteria*: The guidelines incorporate widely recognized tools such as the Beers Criteria and the STOPP/START Criteria, which are used globally to identify PIMs and optimize medication regimens. These tools are adapted to suit the needs of Indian patients, considering regional variations in disease prevalence and medication availability.

- *Patient-centered approaches*: Like international guidelines, these guidelines emphasize the importance of shared decision-making and patient engagement. However, they place particular emphasis on culturally sensitive communication and the inclusion of family members in the decision-making process, reflecting the collectivist nature of Indian society.
- *Focus on affordability and accessibility*: The guidelines address the economic constraints faced by many Indian patients by encouraging the use of cost-effective therapies and promoting access to affordable medications. This focus on affordability distinguishes them from some international frameworks that may not prioritize economic considerations to the same extent.

FUTURE DIRECTIONS

To enhance the effectiveness and applicability of the deprescribing guidelines, several areas for future research and guideline refinement have been identified:

- *Research on long-term outcomes*: While current evidence supports the benefits of deprescribing in reducing adverse events and improving quality of life, more research is needed to evaluate the long-term outcomes of deprescribing interventions, particularly in diverse patient populations and healthcare settings.
- *Development of tailored interventions*: Future research should focus on developing and testing tailored deprescribing interventions that address specific patient characteristics, such as genetic factors, comorbidities, and personal preferences.
- *Integration of technology*: The integration of health information technology, such as EHRs and decision support systems, can enhance the implementation and monitoring of deprescribing practices. Future work should explore the development of user-friendly digital tools that facilitate medication reviews and support shared decision-making.
- *Education and training programs*: Continued investment in education and training programs for healthcare providers is essential to ensure that deprescribing practices are effectively implemented. Future efforts should focus on expanding access to these programs and evaluating their impact on clinical practice.
- *Policy and advocacy efforts*: Engaging policymakers and stakeholders in discussions about the benefits of deprescribing can help drive systemic changes that support its integration into routine care. Advocacy efforts should aim to raise awareness of the importance of medication optimization and the role of deprescribing in improving patient outcomes.
- *Expanding the workforce and sustaining deprescribing efforts*: To implement deprescribing on a larger scale across India's vast elderly population, there is an urgent need to expand the pool of professionals skilled in this area. Currently, trained clinical pharmacologists at the DM and MD Internal Medicine, Geriatric Medicine and Pharmacology trained in CPRRF are limited, and primary care is often delivered by MBBS-trained physicians, alternate medicine specialists, and practitioners with varying levels of expertise.

Enhancing the training and exposure of these groups to deprescribing practices is crucial. Furthermore, sustaining deprescribing efforts requires continuous follow-up to ensure that patients do not revert to inappropriate or redundant medication regimens upon returning to their usual healthcare providers. This calls for establishing mechanisms to monitor deprescribing outcomes and maintain communication across the healthcare continuum to support ongoing medication optimization.

CONCLUSION

Deprescribing is a crucial component of patient-centered care, particularly in India, where the burden of polypharmacy and medication-related harm is significant. The guidelines outlined in this document provide a strategic approach to minimizing the risks associated with inappropriate medication use, ultimately enhancing the quality of life for patients.

By adopting these advices, healthcare providers can reduce the incidence of adverse drug events, improve patient outcomes, and promote a culture of rational prescribing. The focus on patient engagement and shared decision-making empowers patients to take an active role in their healthcare, leading to more personalized and effective treatment plans.

The successful implementation of these deprescribing guidelines has the potential to transform patient care in India, ensuring that medication regimens are both safe and aligned with the health needs and goals of each individual.

This document provides a comprehensive framework for healthcare providers to identify and manage PIMs, ensuring that medication regimens are both safe and effective.

SUMMARY OF KEY POINTS

- *Identification of PIMs*: Utilizing tools such as the Beers Criteria and STOPP/START Criteria, healthcare providers can systematically identify PIMs and reduce the risks associated with polypharmacy. These tools facilitate the optimization of medication regimens, enhancing patient safety, and improving outcomes.
- *Risk assessment*: By evaluating drug-drug and drug-disease interactions, as well as considering cumulative effects and patient-specific factors, healthcare providers can better understand the risks and benefits associated with each medication. This approach ensures that treatment plans are tailored to individual patient needs.
- *Patient-centered approach*: The guidelines emphasize shared decision-making and individualized care planning, fostering greater patient engagement, and satisfaction. By involving patients in their care decisions, healthcare providers can better align treatment goals with patient preferences and values.
- *Prioritization framework*: A structured framework for prioritizing medications for deprescription based on risk and benefit analysis helps ensure that the most appropriate and effective treatments are maintained while minimizing unnecessary medication use.

- *Tapering and monitoring*: Safe tapering protocols and robust monitoring strategies are essential for minimizing withdrawal symptoms and ensuring successful deprescribing. These protocols help healthcare providers manage the transition from high-risk medications to safer alternatives effectively.
- *Implementation strategies*: The integration of tools, educational programs, and strategies to overcome challenges and barriers is vital for the successful implementation of deprescribing practices. By addressing these factors, healthcare providers can ensure that deprescribing becomes a routine part of patient care.

SUGGESTED READINGS

1. Bhagavathula AS, Vidyasagar K, Chhabra M, Rashid M, Sharma R, Bandari DK, et al. Prevalence of Polypharmacy, Hyperpolypharmacy and Potentially Inappropriate Medication Use in Older Adults in India: A Systematic Review and Meta-Analysis. Front Pharmacol. 2021;12:685518.
2. Samajdar SS, Das S, Sarkar S, Mukherjee S, Pathak A, Stålsby Lundborg C, et al. Association between Polypharmacy and Cardiovascular Autonomic Function among Elderly Patients in an Urban Municipality Area of Kolkata, India: A Record-Based Cross-Sectional Study. Geriatrics (Basel). 2022;7(6):136.
3. Balarajan Y, Selvaraj S, Subramanian SV. Health care and equity in India. Lancet. 2011;377:505-15.
4. Porter G, Grills N. Medication misuse in India: a major public health issue in India. J Public Health (Oxf). 2016;3(2):e150-7.
5. Chandy SJ, Thomas K, Mathai E, Antonisamy B, Holloway KA, Stalsby Lundborg C, et al. Patterns of antibiotic use in the community and challenges of antibiotic surveillance in a lower-middle-income country setting: a repeated cross-sectional study in Vellore, south India. J Antimicrob Chemother. 2013;68(1):229-36.
6. Salunkhe SD, Pandit VA, Dawane JS, Sarda KD, More CS. Study of over the counter sale of antimicrobials in pharmacy outlets in Pune, India: a cross sectional study. Int J Pharm Bio Sci. 2013;4(2):616-22.
7. Rathnakar UP, Sharma NK, Garg R, Unnikrishnan B, Krishnahn G. A Study on the Sale of Antimicrobial Agents without Prescriptions in Pharmacies in an Urban Area in South India. J Clin Diagn Res. 2012;6(6):951-4.
8. Hajjar ER, Cafiero AC, Hanlon JT. Polypharmacy in elderly patients. Am J Geriatr Pharmacother. 2007;5(4):345-51.
9. Hopcroft P, Peel NM, Poudel A, Scott IA, Gray LC, Hubbard RE. Prescribing for older people discharged from the acute sector to residential aged-care facilities. Intern Med J. 2014;44(10):1034-7.
10. Todd A, Holmes HM. Recommendations to support deprescribing medications late in life. Int J Clin Pharm. 2015;37(5):678-81.
11. By the 2023 American Geriatrics Society Beers Criteria® Update Expert Panel. American Geriatrics Society 2023 updated AGS Beers Criteria® for potentially inappropriate medication use in older adults. J Am Geriatr Soc. 2023;71(7):2052-81.
12. O'Mahony D, Cherubini A, Guiteras AR, Denkinger M, Beuscart JB, Onder G, et al. STOPP/START criteria for potentially inappropriate prescribing in older people: version 3. Eur Geriatr Med. 2023;14(4):625-32.
13. Scott IA, Hilmer SN, Reeve E, Potter K, Le Couteur D, Rigby D, et al. Reducing inappropriate polypharmacy—the process of deprescribing. JAMA Intern Med. 2015;175:827-34.
14. Samajdar SS, Tripathi SK. Clinical Pharmacological Reconciliation, Review, and Feedback in Ensuring Patient Safety: A Commentary. J Clin Pharmacol. 2023;63(9):1074-5.

15. Samajdar SS, Mukherjee S, Sarkar S, Sen S, Tripathi SK, Joshi SR, et al. Clinical Pharmacological Consultation in Optimizing Diabetic Patient Care: A Cross-sectional Observational Study. Bengal Physician J. 2023;10(1):6-8.
16. Anderson K, Stowasser D, Freeman C, Scott I. Prescriber barriers and enablers to minimising potentially inappropriate medications in adults: a systematic review and thematic synthesis. BMJ Open. 2014;4(12):e006544.
17. Samajdar SS, Mukherjee S, Tripathi SK, Pal J, Joshi S. Deprescribing for Better Patient Outcomes in Chronic Long Term Care and Role of Clinical Pharmacological Review. J Assoc Physicians India. 2021;69(11):11-2.
18. Nishtala PS, Salahudeen MS, Hilmer SN. Anticholinergics: theoretical and clinical overview. Expert Opin Drug Saf. 2016;15(6):753-68.
19. Saha D, Samajdar SS, Begum SA, Mukherjee S, Tripathi SK, Pal J, et al. Anticholinergic burden in geriatric patients attending clinical pharmacology clinic—a descriptive cross-sectional study in Eastern India. J Indian Med Assoc. 2022;120(10):39-43.
20. Taipale HT, Bell JS, Soini H, Pitkälä KH. Sedative load and mortality among residents of long-term care facilities: a prospective cohort study. Drugs Aging. 2009;26(10):871-81.
21. Onder G, Petrovic M, Tangiisuran B, Meinardi MC, Markito-Notenboom WP, Somers A, et al. Development and validation of a score to assess risk of adverse drug reactions among in-hospital patients 65 years or older: the GerontoNet ADR risk score. Arch Intern Med. 2010;170(13):1142-8.
22. Iyer S, Naganathan V, McLachlan AJ, Le Couteur DG. Medication withdrawal trials in people aged 65 years and older: a systematic review. Drugs Aging. 2008;25(12):1021-31.
23. Mistler LA, Mellman TA, Drake RE. A pilot study testing a medication algorithm to reduce polypharmacy. Qual Saf Health Care. 2009;18(1):55-8.
24. Scott IA, Gray LC, Martin JH, Mitchell CA. Minimizing inappropriate medications in older populations: a 10-step conceptual framework. Am J Med. 2012;125(6):529-37.e4.
25. Samajdar SS, Mukherjee S, Sharma J, Pal J, Tripathi SK, Saboo B, et al. Clinical Pharmacological Reconciliation, Review, and Feedback in Elderly Care: A Transformative Approach. J Indian Acad Geriatr. 2024;20(3):150-3.
26. Samajdar SS, Chatterjee N, Pal J, George M, Sarkar S, Sen S, et al. Rational Deprescribing Practices in Elderly Patients: An Expert Opinion. Bengal Physician J. 2024;11(3):133-45.

4

CHAPTER

Drug–Drug Interaction and Adverse Drug Reaction in Elderly

ABSTRACT

Drug–drug interactions (DDIs) and adverse drug reactions (ADRs) are critical concerns in elderly healthcare due to altered pharmacokinetics, multimorbidity, and polypharmacy. DDIs occur when two or more drugs interact, modifying therapeutic effects or increasing the risk of adverse outcomes. This chapter explores the mechanisms of DDIs, including pharmacokinetic and pharmacodynamic interactions, emphasizing the vulnerabilities introduced by age-related physiological changes. Specific examples of detrimental and beneficial DDIs are discussed, highlighting the need for careful prescription practices, especially in the elderly population. Strategies to identify and manage DDIs, including medication reconciliation and the use of advanced decision-support tools, are provided to minimize risks and optimize therapeutic outcomes.

Adverse drug reactions, defined as unintended and harmful drug responses, are significantly prevalent in the elderly due to increased drug sensitivity, polypharmacy, and comorbid conditions. Most ADRs are predictable (type A), linked to dose-dependent effects, and avoidable with appropriate prescribing, while unpredictable (type B) reactions pose additional challenges. The chapter outlines the causes of increased ADR risks in older adults, including physiological changes, cognitive impairments, and frailty. Tools such as the Beers Criteria, STOPP/START (Screening Tool of Older Persons' Potentially Inappropriate Prescriptions/Screening Tool to Alert doctors of Right Treatments) guidelines, and ARMOR framework are recommended for identifying inappropriate prescriptions and preventing ADRs.

Preventive strategies, such as rational prescribing, "start low and go slow" dosing, and Clinical Pharmacological Reconciliation Review and Feedback (CPRRF), are emphasized. Effective management of ADRs involves recognizing adverse events, assessing causality through validated scales, documenting reactions, and reporting to pharmacovigilance systems. By integrating these strategies into clinical practice, the burden of DDIs and ADRs can be significantly reduced, improving patient safety and quality of care for the elderly.

DRUG–DRUG INTERACTION IN ELDERLY

INTRODUCTION

A drug–drug interaction (DDI) is said to happen when two or more drugs interact with each other that modify the response of interacting drug(s). Often such (major) interactions are clinically significant and may have either beneficial effects for the disease condition or detrimental effects such as loss of/decrease in effect or adverse drug reactions (ADRs) including toxicities. For example, the combination of levodopa and carbidopa provides enhanced levels of levodopa, this is by carbidopa-induced prevention of peripheral decarboxylation of levodopa (beneficial effect); on the other hand, when a sedative is taken with antihistamine, it will produce profound sedation (harmful) in elderly. About 10–20% of the ADRs that require hospitalization are due to harmful DDIs. A cross-sectional study in elderly demonstrated that 72.2% of recruited participants were on drugs with potential CYP-mediated DDI. Major DDIs may have a vivid clinical impact on patient safety, especially in elderly due to their variable pharmacokinetics. Therefore, identification and prevention of possible DDIs among prescribed drugs, and their management are crucial in clinical practice.

The drug's response can also be modified by food, addiction (alcohol and smoking), herbal medicine and dietary supplements, various environmental factors, and even other diseases. For example, monoamine oxidase inhibitors (MAO) inhibitors with cheese products will cause a cheese reaction; nasal decongestants in elderly hypertensive patients increase the blood pressure, nonsteroidal anti-inflammatory drugs (NSAIDs) in asthmatic may exacerbate airway obstruction, etc.

MECHANISMS OF DRUG–DRUG INTERACTIONS

Drug–drug interactions can have pharmacokinetic or pharmacodynamic mechanisms. In pharmacokinetic interactions, one drug affects the absorption, distribution, metabolism, or excretion of another drug. Pharmacokinetic DDIs are commonly based on:

- *Altered metabolism:* It is attributable to the effects on cytochrome P450 (CYP450) isoenzymes (most common isoenzyme is CYP3A4, followed by 2C19, 2C9, 1A2, 2E6, and 2D6). Inhibition or induction of such drug-metabolizing isoenzymes may cause clinically important DDIs. The drugs interacting with CYP450 isoenzymes can be classified as substrates, inducers, or inhibitors.
- *Altered excretion:* It is attributable to the effect of altered secretion at proximal convoluted tubule due to competition of drugs at energy-dependent cationic and anionic transport pumps **(Table 1)**. DDI may also alter enterohepatic circulation of the various drugs, especially in elderly due to preexisting age-induced (and laxative abuse) gut microbiota dysbiosis.
- *Displacement of a drug from a protein-binding site by another drug:* This increases the unbound concentration of the displaced drug, which can lead to enhanced pharmacological effects or toxicities.
- *Altered transportation:* Several drugs are substrates of transport-protein-complexes, such as P-glycoprotein (P-gp), OATP1B1, and BRCP; which are

TABLE 1: Examples of some DDIs having detrimental effects.

Enzyme inducer	Enzyme induced	Substrate	Likely interaction and comments
Phenobarbitone, phenytoin, carbamazepine, efavirenz, pioglitazone, and glucocorticoids	CYP3A4	Midazolam, alprazolam, ritonavir, calcium channel blockers, theophylline, and macrolides	• Induction of metabolism → loss of efficacy of substrate drugs • Avoid the concurrent use or increase the dose of substrate drugs with monitoring
Rifampicin and phenobarbitone	CYP3A4 and CYPEC9	Oral contraceptive, warfarin, ibuprofen, tamoxifen, and losartan	
Enzyme inhibitor	**Enzyme inhibited**	**Substrate**	**Likely interaction and comments**
Erythromycin, clarithromycin, ketoconazole, itraconazole, and ritonavir	CYP3A4	Phenytoin, carbamazepine, warfarin, sulfonylureas, diazepam, theophylline, cyclosporine, and statins	• Inhibition of metabolism by CYP3A4 → toxicity of substrate drugs • Avoid concurrent use or readjust the dose of substrate drug
Ciprofloxacin and norfloxacin	Hepatic microsomal mixed function oxidases	Theophylline and warfarin	• Inhibition of metabolism → toxicity of substrate drugs • Monitor and reduce dose of substrate drug

(DDIs: drug–drug interactions)

expressed in hepatocytes, enterocytes, epithelial cells of the renal tubules, the blood–brain barrier, and the placenta. The effects of these transporters are subject to inhibition or induction that can elicit DDIs.

In pharmacodynamic interactions, the two drugs have either additive/summation, synergistic, or antagonistic effects by varied mechanisms (receptor or nonreceptor mediated).

The physiological changes in elderly may pose some extra impact on above-mentioned mechanisms of DDI such as:

- *Reduced renal excretory (secretory) capacity:* Removal of hydrophilic drugs via kidneys may be significantly impaired, which requires adjustment of drug dose.
- *Impaired hepatic metabolism:* Drug metabolism may be affected by age-related changes in liver, such as 20–40% decrease in liver size, 40–60% decrease in blood flow through liver, and 30% decrease in cytochrome P450 (CYP450) oxidase activity in elderly people compared to young adults. So, drugs that are metabolized by liver may require lower or less frequent doses in older people; similarly, prodrugs requiring activation through hepatic metabolism may be less effective in older people.
- *Changes in plasma protein concentration:* The level of albumin is approximately 19% lower in the elderly than in the young population. So, free drug concentration of the albumin-bound drugs may be increased to the potential toxic level, even when the total drug concentration is within the therapeutic

range. In contrast, a slight increase in alpha-1 acid glycoprotein, observed in healthy elderly, but less pronounced in the presence of a disease, may cause an increase in the concentration of some drugs, e.g., propranolol.
- *Lower levels of transporters:* In elderly, the concentration of P-gp transporters in brain and intestinal tissue is lower than in younger people, especially in those suffering from dementia. This may affect the transport of various drugs across the cell membrane.

Changes in drug sensitivity: Pharmacodynamic changes are also associated with aging. For example, age-related decrease in response to agonists and antagonists of beta-adrenoreceptors increases the risk of orthostatic hypotension to antihypertensive drugs and increases sensitivity of central nervous system to opioids, benzodiazepines, and psychotropic drugs in elderly. The examples of some clinically significant DDIs are given in **Tables 1 to 3**.

TABLE 2: Examples of some DDIs having interaction and comments.

Drug altering action of another drug	Drug whose action is altered	Likely interaction and comments
Cyclosporin	Rosuvastatin	Causes sevenfold increase in levels of statin due to inhibition of hepatic sinusoidal OATP1B1 and BRCP transporter
Ampicillin and amoxicillin	Warfarin	Inhibition of gut flora → decreased vitamin K production in gut → risk of bleeding; monitor INR and reduce anticoagulant dose if needed
Iron salts, calcium salts, antacids, and sucralfate	Tetracyclines and fluoroquinolones	Decreased absorption due to formation of complexes in GIT → failure of antibiotic therapy
Furosemide	• Minocycline • Aminoglycoside • Spironolactone	• Enhanced vestibular toxicity; avoid concurrent use • Additive ototoxicity and nephrotoxicity; avoid concurrent use as it increases risk of hyponatremia—the combination of furosemide and spironolactone may increase the risk of hyponatremia, particularly in patients with underlying risk factors like advanced age, renal impairment, or excessive fluid loss
Aspirin and other NSAIDs	Sulfonylureas, phenytoin, valproate, and methotrexate	Displacement and/or reduced elimination → toxicity of object drug; avoid concurrent use; substitute NSAID with paracetamol
	Warfarin and heparin	• Displacement of warfarin • Enhanced risk of bleeding due to additional antiplatelet action and gastric mucosal damage; caution in concurrent use
	ACE inhibitors, beta blockers, thiazide diuretics, and furosemide	Reduced antihypertensive effect due to inhibition of renal PG synthesis; avoid concurrent use

(ACE: angiotensin-converting enzyme; DDIs: drug–drug interactions; GIT: gastrointestinal tract; INR: international normalized ratio; NSAIDs: nonsteroidal anti-inflammatory drugs; PG: prostaglandins)

TABLE 3: Examples of some DDIs having beneficial effects.

Drugs involved	Mechanism	Benefits
Sulfamethoxazole + trimethoprim	Sulfonamides block dihydropteroic acid synthase and trimethoprim blocks dihydrofolate reductase	Individually, drugs are bacteriostatic but combination makes it bactericidal
Ibuprofen/ Aceclofenac + paracetamol	Both act by inhibition of prostaglandin synthesis	Enhanced analgesic effect
Beta-lactam antibiotics + aminoglycosides	Beta-lactam antibiotics inhibit the bacterial cell wall synthesis, which facilitates the passive diffusion of aminoglycosides if given together	Enhanced antimicrobial activity
Ritonavir + lopinavir/ other PIs	Ritonavir is a CYP3A4 inhibitor, so it increases the plasma concentration of other protease inhibitors (PIs)	Improved viral suppression
Probenecid + penicillin/ sulfonamide/ zidovudine	Probenecid competes with penicillin, sulfonamides, and zidovudine for binding to the anionic transporter	Extending the duration of action of penicillin/ sulfonamide/zidovudine
Probenecid + cidofovir	Probenecid decreases both the renal clearance of cidofovir and the incidence of nephrotoxicity by binding to the anionic transporter and blocking its active tubular secretion	Probenecid as a nephron-protectant during cidofovir therapy
ARB + CCB/diuretics	Acts by different mechanism of action	Added antihypertensive effect, reduces the frequency of ankle edema, reduces the chance of hypokalemia

(ARB: angiotensin II receptor blocker; CCB: calcium channel blocker; DDIs: drug–drug interactions)

TYPES OF DRUG–DRUG INTERACTIONS

Interactions between various drugs may be categorized as follows:

- *Behavioral DDI:* It occurs when one drug alters the patient's behavior, so that the compliance for another drug increases. For example, when a depressed patient starts an antidepressant, his/her condition gradually improves, which makes him/her more compliant with other medications.
- *Pharmaceutical DDI:* It occurs when the formulation of one drug is altered by another drug before its administration. For example, precipitation of sodium thiopentone and vecuronium within an intravenous set.
- *Pharmacokinetic DDI:* Such interaction occurs when one drug modifies the pharmacokinetics of another drug. For example, enzyme inducers like phenytoin increase the metabolism of vitamin D leading to osteomalacia and unwanted pregnancy can happen if oral contraceptives are taken concomitantly with rifampicin or phenytoin, etc.

- *Pharmacodynamic DDI:* This type of interaction is seen when two drugs have either additive or synergistic effects leading to an overall increased response or opposing effects leading to an overall decreased response. For example, concurrent use of digitalis and propranolol causes significant bradycardia and central nervous system (CNS) stimulants antagonize the effect of CNS depressants, etc.

RISK FACTORS OF DRUG–DRUG INTERACTIONS

The following conditions may transform a clinically insignificant interaction into a significant one:

- *Acute medical conditions (like dehydration, infection, etc.):* These may alter the pharmacokinetics of the drug(s) such as inhibition of hepatic drug metabolism.
- *Chronic medical conditions:* Elderly patients having compromised renal and/or hepatic function and decrease in clearance may lead to accumulation of drugs or their metabolites.
- Drug(s) with narrow therapeutic index have higher risk for DDI-related side effects.
- Elderly females have reduced metabolic capacity as compared to males.
- Polypharmacy increases the risk of pharmacokinetic and/or pharmacodynamic DDIs.
- Pharmacogenetic characteristics alter the metabolic capacity (ultrarapid or poor metabolizers), which may cause rapid and complete metabolism of drug and increase concentration of drug metabolites or accumulation of drugs.

MEASURES TO AVOID UNWANTED DRUG–DRUG INTERACTIONS IN CLINICAL PRACTICE

As discussed earlier, DDIs could have beneficial or detrimental effects. Certainly, those beneficial interactions can be used for optimum therapeutic response and at the same time harmful DDIs should be avoided. A rational prescription should contain least and only clinically insignificant harmful DDI. The *10 "rules"* to prevent and manage potential DDIs in clinical practice are:

1. *Elicit detailed drug history:* This will help in identifying if the present complaint is due to any DDI-related ADR (drug-induced disease) of ongoing therapy or a new disease entity. This will also help in prescribing new drug(s) that are compatible with existing therapy. The detailed drug history should include prescription and nonprescription medicines, over-the-counter medicines, herbal medicine, and dietary supplements.
2. *Medication reconciliation:* If any DDI between the existing drugs has been identified (occurred), then reconcile it with the best suitable alternative.
3. *Updated and thorough pharmacological knowledge*: Prescribe the drugs that are well known, especially related to the pharmacokinetics and pharmacodynamics of the drugs.
4. *Check the prescribing information (or package insert):* Never hesitate to read and learn, especially the drug safety and potential DDI section of the

prescribing information, if the clinical pharmacology of the drug is not well known.

5. *Update about drug alert:* The regulatory authority of the country [Drugs Controller General of India (DCGI), US Food and Drug Administration (US FDA), etc.] often issues alerts for healthcare professionals. For example, in 2009, FDA issued an alert on potential interactions between clopidogrel and omeprazole that should not be taken together. The Global Patient Safety Alert is a website that has a collection of alerts, advisories, and recommendations about patient safety.
6. *Avoid drugs with a narrow therapeutic index:* Avoid those drugs if not absolutely essential. As they are more susceptible to DDIs-related adverse effects.
7. *Avoid polypharmacy:* It is a potential risk factor for DDIs.
8. *Consider patients' (altered) physiology during prescribing:* That may allow easy recognition of possible and potential DDIs-induced ADR.
9. *Electronic software-based drug interaction checker:*
    a. *Computerized Physician Order Entry (CPOE) with Clinical Decision Support Systems (CDSSs):* CPOE is also called an electronic prescribing system or e-prescribing with CDSS, which aims to check the medication errors, DDIs, and drug allergies. The CDSS or clinical decision support (CDS) helps in improving the physician decisions by alerts, suggestions, and reminders.
    b. *Installation of software systems:* There are some free and low-cost software systems available to identify potential DDIs. These electronic programs are helpful in lowering the risk and adverse effects due to interactions. Such software are:
        i. Epocrates Rx http://www.epocrates.com/ products/rx/
        ii. https://www.drugs.com/drug_interactions.html
        iii. eRx http://www.nationalerx.com/ (National ePrescribing Patient Safety Initiative)
        iv. GeneMedRx http://www.genemedrx.com/providerinfo.php (drug-drug and drug-gene interactions)
        v. https://www.skyscape.com/estore/productdetail.aspx?ProductId=431
    c. *Detection of DDIs mediated by CYP enzymes:* Many DDIs occur due to the inhibition or induction of the cytochrome P450 enzymes. This has led to formation of a comprehensive database on cytochrome P450 enzymes known as *"Super CYP"* and development of some software methods that are helpful to predict clinically relevant DDIs. This software allows the users to enter names of different drugs and check their interactions. In addition, it will also provide alternative drug options. For example, omeprazole and nebivolol interact on the CYP level. Omeprazole has an inhibitory effect on CYP2D6 while nebivolol is a substrate. So, to avoid this interaction, omeprazole can be substituted with pantoprazole to get a better response without any adverse effects.
10. *Wise monitoring plan:* If the prescribed regimen contains inevitable DDI, then closely monitor the patient for any ADR, toxicity, or loss of efficacy as a part of augmented routine care. In successive visit, any changes in symptoms,

biomarkers of drug effects, or drug concentrations soon after initiation of treatment will help in identifying DDIs early and can reduce harm. And then, decide accordingly based on the patient's clinical condition.

CONCLUSION

In clinical practice, prescription often contain harmful DDIs. Likewise, clinicians often encounter patients presented with mild-to-serious ADRs due to DDI. The altered physiology of the elderly and often inevitable polypharmacy make them vulnerable to the unwanted DDI. The common and most potential DDI can be identified by applying principles of clinical pharmacology. In addition, increased vigilance by clinicians during prescription also improves the chances of identifying unwanted DDI before they can cause significant harm. The prescribed drugs should be well-known and judiciously prescribed. With the availability of computerized prescriptions and various software for detection of DDIs, it has now become easier for the clinicians to select the right drugs and dosage that will prevent DDIs.

ADVERSE DRUG REACTIONS IN ELDERLY

INTRODUCTION

World Health Organization (WHO) defines an ADR as *"any response to a drug which is noxious and unintended, and which occurs at doses normally used in man for prophylaxis, diagnosis, or therapy of disease, or for the modification of physiological function."* ADR is an inherent risk of drug use. The frequency of its occurrence and the intensity of harm to the recipient depends on several factors such as the drug used, the regimen prescribed, pharmacokinetics, and genotype of the recipient. ADRs are a major global problem in terms of patient safety and increased cost of the treatment, due to increased chance of hospitalization, prolongation of hospital stays, and additional clinical investigations. Additionally, an ADR may be recognized as a new disease entity that triggers prescription cascades, i.e., new medicine(s) are prescribed for a new disease (ADR) that is a consequence of another medicine.

Adverse drug reactions affect all age groups but the older population is most vulnerable. Previous studies from around the world already established a definite positive correlation between increasing age and ADR rate. Polypharmacy is common in elderly due to multiple comorbidities, and consequently, there is increase the risk of ADRs. Studies conducted in Europe and USA showed the incidence of ADRs in elderly was 42.45% and 54.18%, respectively. Various studies performed in India showed the prevalence of ADR-related hospital admissions was 5.9–16.5% and around 18,000 bed days in each time would be due to ADRs in elderly.

NATURE OF ADVERSE DRUG REACTIONS IN ELDERLY

Rawlins and Thompson classify ADR into two major subtypes: *"Type-A reactions"*, which are dose-dependent and predictable, i.e., related to the known pharmacological effects of the drug, and "*type-B reaction*", which are unpredictable, bizarre in nature or idiosyncratic reaction, i.e., not related to the known pharmacological effects of the drug. Most of the ADRs (80%) are type-A reactions, which are predictable and potentially avoidable too. Type-B ADRs are usually uncommon, but sometimes serious.

The class of drugs most likely to cause type-A reactions in the elderly include antibiotics, anticoagulants, digoxin, diuretics, hypoglycemic agents, antihypertensives, antineoplastic agents, and nonsteroidal anti-inflammatory drugs (NSAIDs). These are responsible for 60% of ADRs leading to hospital admission and 70% of ADRs occurring in hospital. Therefore, ADRs in elderly are largely contributed by medication errors. So, consideration of altered drug disposition and increased pharmacodynamic sensitivity to certain drugs of the elderly should be considered wisely during prescribing.

CAUSES OF INCREASED RISKS OF ADVERSE DRUG REACTIONS IN ELDERLY

As stated earlier, elderly people are more prone to developing ADRs. Age-related physiological changes and affected homeostasis increase the risk of ADRs in elderly. Several factors responsible for increasing the risk of ADRs in elderly are:

- *Altered pharmacokinetics:* Altered pharmacokinetic profile in elderly often increases drug responsiveness and the risk of ADRs. Alterations in absorption (due to reduction in gastric acid secretion, gastrointestinal motility, intestinal surface for absorption, and splanchnic circulation), drug transporter (such as reduction in P-glycoprotein transporter); volumes of drug distributions (decrease in total body water and increase in body fat that can increase the half-life of certain drug), drug metabolism (such as 40–60% decrease in blood flow through liver and 30% decrease in CYP450 oxidase activity and drug interaction due to polypharmacy), and excretion (removal of hydrophilic drugs via kidneys is impaired) in elderly are responsible for higher risk of ADRs.
- *Geriatric syndromes:* Geriatric syndromes, such as falls, delirium, cognitive impairment, orthostatic hypotension, incontinence, and chronic pain, not only reduce the potential benefit of an even rationally chosen drug but also increase the risk of ADRs and at the same time, initiate prescription cascade. For example, antihypertensive drugs can worsen orthostatic hypotension; elderly are more prone to hypoglycemia due to oral antidiabetics; sedative, antiepileptics, opioids, and antidepressants increase the risk of delirium and risk of falls; anticholinergics worsen urinary retention, visual impairments, confusion, delirium, cognitive impairments, and risk of fall; anticoagulant and antiplatelets increase risk of major bleeding; and various drugs have been associated with urinary incontinence, etc.

  Frailty is a geriatric syndrome (affects 5–17% of older adults) of increased vulnerability to stressors that lead to adverse health outcomes. This is due to age-related decline in physiological function and homeostasis across multiorgan systems. Symptoms of frailty include generalized weakness, exhaustion, slow gait, poor balance, decreased physical activity, cognitive impairment, and weight loss. Frail elderly are at increased risk of falls, disability, hospitalizations, and death. Frailty has a significant impact on the development of clinically significant ADRs.

- *Multimorbidity and drug-disease interaction:* The prevalence of multimorbidity (i.e., two or more coexisting chronic diseases) increases with age. Several studies established that multimorbid elderly are at higher risk of developing ADRs or more precisely drug-induced disease. This can be explained as DDI, i.e., when a drug that is used to treat one medical condition exacerbates another underlying medical condition (beta-blockers can worsen asthma symptoms; metoclopramide used for gastric dysmotility can worsen motor symptoms of Parkinson's disease) or the existing condition (such as kidney and liver disease) that can alter drugs' metabolism used for another medical condition.
- *Polypharmacy and DDIs:* Older adults often undergo polypharmacy due to multimorbidity. Global data suggest that >60% older adults receive 5 or more drugs concomitantly. Polypharmacy increases the risk of ADRs. Studies have shown that ADR-related hospitalizations rate is related to the total number of drugs used per day. Polypharmacy-related increase rate of ADRs is often because of the increase in DDI and drug-disease interactions. Data suggests that concomitant use of two medicines has 13% risk of developing ADRs, which increases up to 58–82% when using 5 and 7 or more medicines per day, respectively.
- *Cognitive and sensory impairment vis-à-vis treatment nonadherence:* Cognitive impairment (memory loss, decline in intellectual function, and impaired judgment and decision-making capacity), mental illness, and functional deficits (such as poor vision, instability, or tremor) in elderly have a huge impact on treatment outcome. These are the possible reasons for medication (patient) errors, nonadherence to treatment plans, inappropriate self-medication, development of ADRs, and most importantly underreporting of ADRs. A study on 30,000 elderly people showed that 23.5% of all ADRs were attributed to patient errors.

STRATEGIES TO PREVENT ADVERSE DRUG REACTIONS IN ELDERLY

Various strategies can be adopted by the prescribers to prevent or reduce predictable ADRs in elderly.

- *Appropriate clinical decision-making in diagnosing and rational prescribing:* After diagnosing the certain medical condition(s), prescribers should choose the most suitable drug for the disease condition(s) for the given patient. Then, prescribers should carefully balance the overall benefit against the anticipated risk of each drug.
- *Special considerations in elderly:*
    - Use drugs that have a wide therapeutic window.
    - For a new medicine, "start low and go slow" in dosing whenever possible.
    - When already in polypharmacy, better avoid starting two new medicines at the same time.

- *Updated and thorough pharmacological knowledge:* Prescribe the drugs that are well known, especially related to the pharmacokinetics and pharmacodynamics of the drugs.
- *Avoid polypharmacy:* Decrease in drug burden optimizes the treatment outcome. It reduces ADRs, drug–drug interaction, drug–disease interaction, and cost burden and improves the treatment adherence.
- *Consider age-related physiological changes, decline in organ function, alerted pharmacokinetics, and pharmacodynamic during prescribing:* It will improve treatment outcome and reduce ADRs.
- *Consider age-related cognitive impairment (memory loss, decline in intellectual function, impaired judgment, and decisions-making capacity), mental illness, and functional deficits (such as poor vision, instability, or tremor) in elderly during prescribing:* Choose the appropriate dosage form and regimen to reduce medication errors and to improve treatment adherence and outcome.
- *Prescription reconciliation and Clinical pharmacological reconciliation review and feedback (CPRRF):* These are stepwise processes to generate most appropriate prescription for a given patient at transition of care. The process relies on reviewing and analyzing all previously ongoing and currently required treatment, followed by adjusting the therapy, communicating the same with the patient and the caregivers, and then monitoring the patient at appropriate intervals for assessing the outcome or feedback. In this process, medicine(s) are carefully evaluated for benefit and risk and inappropriate medicine is deprescribed under the supervision. This process reduces the medication error of omission, commission, and duplication.
- *Avoid prescription cascade as far as possible*: The prescribing cascade happens when an additional medication is prescribed to treat an ADR, which is wrongly interpreted as a new medical condition. In such cases, reconcile the treatment with decrease in the current dose or discontinuation of the culprit drug or substitution of the drug with best possible alternative that has lesser ADR. Sometimes prescription cascade becomes inevitable, e.g., use of anti-Parkinson drugs to treat motor symptoms related to long-lasting typical antipsychotic therapy or use of antipsychotics in anti-Parkinson drugs-induced psychosis.
- *Use tools to identify inappropriate prescribing:* Several tools have been developed to identify inappropriate treatment for preventing ADRs in elderly. These are:
    - *The American Geriatrics Society (AGS) Beer's criteria:* This is intended to reduce the exposure of elderly population to potentially inappropriate medications by improving medication selection. It comprises drugs and the drug classes that are potentially inappropriate for use in older adults. Since 1991, it was updated at regular intervals and came with seventh overall update in 2023.
    - *STOPP criteria:* It is comprised of 65 clinically significant criteria with brief explanation for potentially inappropriate prescribing in elderly.
    - *START criteria:* It comprises 22 indicators of potentially important prescribing omissions in elderly.

- *Anticholinergic Cognitive Burden (ACB) scales:* This scale categorizes drugs based on their potential anticholinergic activity with ABC scores ranging from 0–3 (no, mild, moderate, and severe anticholinergic activity, respectively). The ACB Scale identifies 88 medicines with known anticholinergic activity, e.g., amitriptyline (ABC score 3), nortriptyline (score 2), and paroxetine (score 1), etc. The anticholinergic effect in elderly has multiple negative impacts such as urinary retention, drowsiness, confusion, delirium, cognitive impairment, increased risk of fall and mortality, etc. The cumulative ACB score of 3 or more of prescribed drugs is associated with cognitive impairment, increased risk of fall, and mortality. In such cases, the best possible alternative should be chosen to reduce the ADR.
- *Assess, Review, Minimize, Optimize, and Reassess (ARMOR):* It is a stepwise process intended to address and minimize the risk of possible DDIs and ADRs by eliminating nonessential medications and considering patient's clinical profile, altered physiology, and functional status. This is an approach to rationalize polypharmacy, especially in elderly in a systematic and organized process:
  - *A:* Assess the individual for total number of medications and for certain groups of medications that have potential for adverse outcomes.
  - *R:* Review for possible DDIs, drug–disease interactions, drug–body interactions, and ADRs
  - *M:* Minimize nonessential medications and eliminate medications that clearly lack evidence for their usage
  - *O:* Optimize by addressing duplication, redundancy, and adjusting dose based on glomerular filtration rate (GFR), clearance, and other pharmacokinetic parameters.
  - *R:* Reassess heart rate, blood pressure (postural), oxygen saturation rate (>92%) at rest, and activity. Also, reassess functional, cognitive, and clinical status as well as medication adherence.
- *Fit fOR The Aged (FORTA) list:* It represents a list of drugs that have been prepared to guide rational pharmacotherapy in older adults with the aim of reducing the risk of medication error and ADRs. Depending on safety and efficacy, the drugs are classified as:
  - *A (A-bsolutely)* when are indispensable
  - *B (B-eneficial)* when are certainly beneficial
  - *C (C-areful)* when their use is questionable
  - *D (D-o not)* when the prescription of a given drug is avoidable

- *Software to identify potentially inappropriate prescriptions:* Different computer software has been developed to provide support to the prescribers at the time of the prescription, reduce ADRs, and improve outcomes.
  - *Clinical Decisions Support System (CDSS) and Computerized Prescription Support System (CPSS):* This software can identify potentially inappropriate prescriptions (including inappropriate dose and contraindicated treatments), risk of ADRs, and drug interactions.
  - *Computerized Provider Order Entry Systems (CPOE):* This software can detect and avoid possible medication errors.

- *Involve patients and their caregivers in the treatment process by appropriate communication:* The patient and caregiver should be communicated properly about the prescribed treatment and any changes in ongoing drug therapy; provided education about the use of self-medication, over-the-counter drugs, herbal medications, and dietary supplements that can interact with prescribed medications; provided information about the possible ADRs that should be reported, till the limit that will not scare the patient to withhold the treatment.
- *Make an appropriate monitoring plan:* Set up a monitoring plan during prescribing (e.g., visit every 4 weeks) to monitor for intended benefit, failure of treatment, development of any anticipated ADRs (to be detected clinically and/or appropriate laboratory testing), and medication adherence especially in multimorbid patients on polypharmacy.

IDENTIFICATION, MANAGEMENT, AND REPORTING OF ADVERSE DRUG REACTIONS

It is the five-step process:

1. Identifying/recognizing ADRs
2. Treat the patient
3. Assessing causality between drug and suspected reaction by using WHO-UMC causality assessment system or Naranjo ADR Probability scale
4. Documentation of ADR in patient's medical records
5. Reporting ADRs to pharmacovigilance center

Identifying/Recognizing an Adverse Drug Reaction

It is sometimes difficult to identify ADRs due to following reasons:

- Older patients may not report the problem to the doctor (as discussed earlier).
- Prescriber may not be aware of such ADRs.
- ADR can be taken as a new disease/additional clinical feature of the disease being treated.
- Sometimes, it is impossible to distinguish between the disease being treated and the ADR (both drug and disease may act through the same physiological or pathological pathways, e.g., arrythmias due to antiarrhythmic drugs).
- Atypical presentations of an ADR in elderly people may be difficult to identify.

However, a high index of suspicion in older patients (especially those on polypharmacy or having cognitive impairment) and the following systematic approach may be helpful in identifying possible ADRs.

History Vis-à-vis Clinical and Pharmacological Knowledge

For follow-up of the patient, following points should be kept in mind:

- Make sure the medicines ordered and medicines received are the same.
- Confirm whether the medicine is taken by the patient or not.
- If yes, then if the medicine was taken at the dose advised or not.
- Confirm if the present symptoms (new medical problem) appear after the start of new medicine or change the dosage of an ongoing medicine.

For a new patient, the following points should be kept in mind:

- A full medical history and drug history should be taken.
- If possible, inspect and analyze all medicines taken by the patient (to identify error and other nonprescription medicines that the patient is taking, including over-the-counter medicines or traditional medicines including herbal preparations).
- An ADR (or drug-induced disease) should always be one of the differential diagnoses.

Then the prescriber should use his/her clinical and pharmacological knowledge to evaluate if this ADR can be explained by any other cause, e.g., patient's underlying disease, other nonprescription medicines, toxins or foods, etc., patient is taking.

Try to Establish Temporal (Time) Relationships by Answering the Following Question

Does the ADR occur following the medicine administration (immediately or after continuous use)?

Perform thorough Physical Examination and Appropriate Laboratory Investigations if Necessary

- Thorough systemic examination and necessary, lab investigations should be performed whenever required to decide what is the actual cause of this new medical problem (ADR or a new disease).
- The reaction (or new medical problem) should be described clearly and wherever possible, an accurate diagnosis should be provided (e.g., drug-induced extrapyramidal syndrome or fixed drug eruption, etc.).
- Examination, investigation, and accurate diagnosis are also important for providing appropriate management of this present condition.

Always consider the new medical problem as an ADR, when it is well explained by the drug(s) patient is taking or when any other possibility (or disease) is not explaining the patient's new medical condition.

The Effect of Dechallenge and Rechallenge should be Determined

- *Dechallenge (withdrawal of the suspected medicine):* Positive dechallenge is the improvement/resolution of ADR when the suspected medicine is withdrawn. It is a strong, though not conclusive indication of medicine-induced reaction (ADR).
- *Rechallenge (reintroducing the suspected medicine after a dechallenge):* It is only justifiable when the benefit of reintroducing the suspected medicine to the patient outweighs the risk of recurrence of the reaction, which is rare. In some cases, the reaction may be more severe on repeated exposure. Rechallenge requires serious ethical considerations. Positive rechallenge is a conclusive indication of medicine-induced reaction (ADR).

Check the Clinical Pharmacology of the Drug from Authentic Source

Check if the ADR (or new medical problem) is documented to occur with the drug(s) the patient is taking at clinical pharmacology section of package insert or in any other published literature. Note that any documentation does not exclude the possibility of being an ADR. Also, check if the pharmacokinetic or pharmacodynamic properties of the drug(s) scientifically justify such ADR.

Treat the Patient

The promptness and measures to be taken to manage ADR depend on:

- Type of ADR
- Severity of ADR
- Primary disease for which drug was advised
- Patient's clinical condition (comorbidities and organ functions)

Common methods of management include:

- Withdrawal of the suspected drug
- Rescue treatment if necessary. It depends on the type of ADR and its severity.
- Use safer alternatives if available, for primary disease.
- For life-threatening ADR [anaphylaxis, Stevens-Johnson syndrome (SJS), or toxic epidermal necrolysis (TEN)], hospitalization of patient is required.
- If no safer alternative is available or alternative option is inferior to first-line drug (that causes ADR), then decide wisely depending on the situation (severity of primary disease, severity of ADR, etc.). Drug desensitization is often done in this situation.

Assessing Causality between Drug and ADR by Using WHO–Uppsala Monitoring Centre (UMC) Causality Assessment System or Naranjo ADR Probability Scale

It is essential to identify the ADR, assess it, and then establish a causal relationship between the drug and the ADR. There are various causality assessment methods available, which are based on questionnaires and algorithms to evaluate the relationship between a drug and ADR. But amongst them, two most widely accepted and followed are the causality assessment scales proposed by WHO, in collaboration with the Uppsala Monitoring Centre (WHO-UMC scale) and the Naranjo probability scale. These two scales are well structured, transparent, and easy to apply causality assessment methods. **Table 4** summarizes the WHO-UMC causality categories and **Table 5** depicts Naranjo ADR probability scale—items and score.

Documentation of Adverse Drug Reaction in Patient's Medical Records

Every prescriber and hospital should document the ADRs (the drug, the reaction, and how it is treated) in patient's medical records and alert the patient that he/she should always provide such documents to every prescriber on each future visit. This step will prevent future harm to the patient and will shield the prescriber from any legal complications too.

Reporting an Adverse Drug Reaction to Pharmacovigilance Center

What to Report?

All adverse events should be reported.

TABLE 4: The World Health Organization–Uppsala Monitoring Centre (WHO–UMC) causality categories.

Causality term	Assessment criteria
Certain	• Event or laboratory test abnormality, with plausible time relationship to drug intake • Cannot be explained by disease or other drugs • Response to withdrawal plausible (pharmacologically and pathologically) • Event definitive pharmacologically or phenomenologically (i.e., an objective and specific medical disorder or a recognized pharmacologic phenomenon) • Rechallenge satisfactory, if necessary
Probable/Likely	• Event or laboratory test abnormality, with reasonable time relationship to drug intake • Unlikely to be attributed to disease or other drugs • Response to withdrawal clinically reasonable • Rechallenge not required
Possible	• Event or laboratory test abnormality, with reasonable time relationship to drug intake • Could also be explained by disease or other drugs • Information on drug withdrawal may be lacking or unclear
Unlikely	• Event or laboratory test abnormality, with a time relationship - temporal relationship to drug intake that makes a relationship improbable (but not impossible) • Disease or other drugs provide plausible explanation
Conditional/ Unclassified	• Event or laboratory test abnormality • More data for proper assessment is needed or additional data under examination
Unassessable/ Unclassified	• Report suggesting an adverse reaction • Cannot be judged because information is insufficient or contradictory

A reaction is serious when the patient's outcome is:

- Death
- Life-threatening
- Hospitalization (initial or prolonged)
- Disability (significant, persistent, or permanent)
- Congenital anomaly
- Required intervention to prevent permanent impairment or damage

Report nonserious, known or unknown, frequent, or rare ADRs due to medicines, vaccines, herbal products, etc.

Note: Adverse event following immunization (AEFI) can also be reported in serious cases. Notification form available on http://www.ipc.gov.in.

Who can Report?

All healthcare professionals (clinicians, dentists, pharmacists, and nurses, etc.) can report ADRs. Consumers can also fill up the "medicine side-effect reporting form" by themselves.

TABLE 5: Naranjo adverse drug reaction (ADR) probability scale—items and score.

Question	Yes	No	Do not know	Score
1. Are there previous conclusive reports on this reaction?	+1	0	0	
2. Did the adverse event appear after the suspected drug was administered?	+2	−1	0	
3. Did the adverse event improve when the drug was discontinued or a specific antagonist was administered?	+1	0	0	
4. Did the adverse event reappear when the drug was readministered?	+2	−1	0	
5. Are there alternative causes that could on their own have caused the reaction?	−1	+2	0	
6. Did the reaction reappear when a placebo was given?	−1	+1	0	
7. Was the drug detected in blood or other fluids in concentrations known to be toxic?	+1	0	0	
8. Was the reaction more severe when the dose was increased or less severe when the dose was decreased?	+1	0	0	
9. Did the patient have a similar reaction to the same increased dose or less severe when the dose was decreased?	+1	0	0	
10. Was the adverse event confirmed by any objective evidence?	+1	0	0	
Scoring of Naranjo algorithm: >9 = definite ADR; 5–8 = probable ADR; 1–4 = possible ADR; 0 = doubtful ADR			Total score:	

Source: Naranjo et al. (1981).

Where to Report?

- Duly filled-in suspected ADR reporting form can be sent to the nearest ADR Monitoring Centre (AMC) or directly to the National Coordination Centre (NCC) for Pharmacovigilance Programme of India (PvPI).
- Call on Helpline (Toll Free) 1800 180 3024 to report ADRs or directly mail this filled form to pvpi.ipc@gov.in
- A list of nationwide AMCs is available at: http://www.ipc.gov.in, http://www.ipc.gov.in/PvPI/pv_home.html

What Happens to the Submitted Information?

- Information provided in this form is handled in strict confidence. The causality assessment is carried out at AMCs by using WHO-UMC scale. The analyzed forms are forwarded to the NCC through ADR database. Finally, the data is analyzed and forwarded to the Global Pharmacovigilance Database managed by WHO-UMC in Sweden.
- The reports are periodically reviewed by the NCC-PvPI. The information generated on the basis of these reports helps in continuous assessment of the benefit-risk ratio of medicines.

- The information is submitted to the steering committee of PvPI constituted by the Ministry of Health and Family Welfare. The Committee is entrusted with the responsibility to review the data and suggest any interventions that may be required.

Mandatory Fields for Suspected Adverse Drug Reaction Reporting Form

- Patient initials
- Age at onset of reaction
- Reaction term(s)
- Date of onset of reaction
- Suspected medication(s)
- Reporter information

CONCLUSION

Medicines are crucial to treat acute or chronic illness, alleviate pain, and improve the quality of life in geriatric healthcare. As the age advances, there are changes in drug disposition and pharmacodynamic responses, which have significant clinical impact. In addition, polypharmacy, multimorbidity, and frailty in elderly raise the risk of ADRs. Therefore, a holistic approach is required for this vulnerable population. Appropriate clinical decision-making in diagnosing and rational prescribing play a major role in prevention of ADRs in elderly. Several tools have been developed to identify inappropriate treatment and some computer software are available to provide support to the prescribers at the time of the prescription, which reduce ADRs and improve outcomes. But despite these tools, preventing ADRs in elderly is still very challenging. Approaches focusing on pharmaceutical principles like medication review, prescription reconciliation, and CPRRF should be used to reduce the burden of ADRs, keeping in mind patients' characteristics, needs, and health priorities.

SUGGESTED READINGS

1. World Health Organization. (2002). Safety of Medicines: A guide to detecting and reporting adverse drug reactions. [online] Available from https://iris.who.int/bitstream/handle/10665/67378/WHO_EDM_QSM_2002.2.pdf?sequence=1 [Last accessed January, 2025].
2. World Health Organization. (2013). The Use of the WHO–UMC system for standardized Case Causality Assessment. [online] Available from https://www.who.int/publications/m/item/WHO-causality-assessment [Last accessed January, 2025].
3. Indian Pharmacopoeia Commission (National Coordination Centre–Pharmacovigilance Programme of India). 2024. Suspected Adverse Drug Reaction Reporting Form. [online] Available from https://cdsco.gov.in/opencms/export/sites/CDSCO_WEB/Pdfdocuments/Consumer_Section_PDFs/ADRRF_2.pdf [Last accessed January, 2025].
4. Indian Pharmacopoeia Commission. (2023). ADR Reporting tools. [online] Available from https://ipc.gov.in/mandates/pvpi/adr-reporting.html [Last accessed January, 2025].
5. Naranjo CA, Busto U, Sellers EM, Sandor P, Ruiz I, Roberts EA, et al. A method for estimating the probability of adverse drug reactions. Clin Pharmacol Ther. 1981;30(2):239-45.
6. By the 2023 American Geriatrics Society Beers Criteria® Update Expert Panel. American Geriatrics Society 2023 updated AGS Beers Criteria® for potentially inappropriate medication use in older adults. J Am Geriatr Soc. 2023;71(7):2052-81.

7. O'Mahony D, Cherubini A, Guiteras AR, Denkinger M, Beuscart JB, Onder G, et al. STOPP/START criteria for potentially inappropriate prescribing in older people: Version 3. Eur Geriatr Med. 2023;14(4):625-32. Erratum in: Eur Geriatr Med. 2023;14(4):633
8. Aliouche H. (2025). What is the anticholinergic cognitive burden scale? [online] Available from https://www.news-medical.net/health/What-is-the-Anticholinergic-Cognitive-Burden-Scale.aspx [Last accessed January, 2025].
9. Haque R. ARMOR: A Tool to Evaluate Polypharmacy in Elderly Persons. ALTC. 2009:2-6.
10. Pazan F, Weiss C, Wehling M; FORTA. The FORTA (Fit fOR The Aged) List 2021: Fourth Version of a Validated Clinical Aid for Improved Pharmacotherapy in Older Adults. Drugs Aging. 2022;39(3):245-7. Erratum in: Drugs Aging. 2022;39(6):485.
11. Samajdar SS, Tripathi SK. Clinical pharmacological reconciliation, review, and feedback in ensuring patient safety: A Commentary. J Clin Pharmacol. 2023;63(9):1074-5.
12. Gujjarlamudi HB. Polytherapy and drug interactions in elderly. J Midlife Health. 2016;7(3):105-7.
13. Błeszyńska E, Wierucki Ł, Zdrojewski T, Renke M. Pharmacological interactions in the elderly. Medicina (Kaunas). 2020;56(7):320.
14. AL-Musawe L, Torre C, Guerreiro JP, Rodrigues AT, Raposo JF, Mota-Filipe H, et al. Polypharmacy, potentially serious clinically relevant drug-drug interactions, and inappropriate medicines in elderly people with type 2 diabetes and their impact on quality of life. Pharm Res Perspect. 2020;8(4):e00621
15. Snyder BD, Polasek TM, Doogue MP. Drug Interactions: Principles and Practice. Austr Prescr. 2012;35:85-8.
16. Muhammad KR. Potential drug-drug interactions and strategies for their detection and prevention. Farmacia. 2019;67:572-9.
17. Grattagliano I, Portincasa P, D'Ambrosio G, Palmieri VO, Palasciano G. Avoiding drug interactions: Here's help. J Fam Prac. 2010;59:322-9.
18. Corie K, Hardmann JG. Mechanisms of drug interactions: pharmacodynamics and pharmacokinetics. Anaest & Int Care Med. 2014;15(7):305-8.
19. Zazzara MB, Palmer K, Vetrano DL, Carfì A, Onder G. Adverse drug reactions in older adults: A narrative review of the literature. Eur Geriatr Med. 2021;12(3):463-73. Erratum in: Eur Geriatr Med. 2022;13(1):307.
20. Pretorius RW, Gataric G, Swedlund SK, Miller JR. Reducing the risk of adverse drug events in older adults. Am Fam Physician. 2013;87(5):331-6.
21. Won SH, Suh SY, Yim E, Ahn HY. Risk factors related to serious adverse drug reactions reported through electronic submission during hospitalization in elderly patients. Korean J Fam Med. 2022;43(2):125-31.
22. Davies EA, O'Mahony MS. Adverse drug reactions in special populations-theelderly. Br J Clin Pharmacol. 2015;80(4):796-807.
23. Yadesa TM, Kitutu FE, Deyno S, Ogwang PE, Tamukong R, Alele PE. Prevalence, characteristics and predicting risk factors of adverse drug reactions among hospitalized older adults: A systematic review and meta-analysis. SAGE Open Medicine. 2021;9.
24. Hilmer SN, McLachlan AJ, Le Couteur DG. Clinical pharmacology in the geriatric patient. Fund Clin Pharmacol. 2007;21(3):217-30.
25. Hughes JE, Moriarty F, Bennett KE, Cahir C. Drug-drug interactions and the risk of adverse drug reaction-related hospital admissions in the older population. Br J Clinical pharmacol. 2023;90(4):959-75.
26. Cahir C, Bennett K, Teljeur C, Fahey T. Potentially inappropriate prescribing and adverse health outcomes in community dwelling older patients. Br J Clin Pharmacol. 2014;77(1):201-10.

5

CHAPTER

Criteria and Tools for Rational Prescribing

ABSTRACT

The growing global elderly population has led to an increased prevalence of polypharmacy, placing older adults at heightened risk of adverse drug reactions (ADRs) and inappropriate prescribing. This chapter explores various tools and criteria designed to promote rational prescribing practices in geriatric care, emphasizing their role in improving medication safety and optimizing therapeutic outcomes.

Explicit criteria, such as the American Geriatrics Society (AGS) Beers Criteria, STOPP/START criteria, and FORTA system, provide evidence-based guidelines for identifying potentially inappropriate medications (PIMs) and prescribing omissions. Implicit tools like the Medication Appropriateness Index (MAI) leverage clinical judgment for evaluating therapeutic appropriateness, addressing aspects often overlooked by criterion-based approaches. Mixed methodologies, including tools such as ARMOR and TIMER, integrate both explicit and implicit elements, offering comprehensive frameworks for medication assessment.

Recent innovations, such as digital platforms like the "Fast&Rational" web app, leverage artificial intelligence to streamline the application of these tools, enabling efficient and patient-specific evaluations. However, challenges remain in routine implementation, including limited access to resources, barriers to deprescribing, and variability in physician practices, particularly in India. Indian studies reveal high rates of polypharmacy and PIM use among the elderly, underscoring the urgent need for greater adoption of these tools to reduce ADRs and enhance clinical outcomes.

The chapter emphasizes the importance of individualized care, where decisions to initiate, adjust, or discontinue medications consider the patient's health conditions, life expectancy, and treatment goals. A holistic approach combining updated criteria, advanced technologies, and shared decision-making is essential for addressing the complexities of geriatric prescribing and ensuring safer, more effective care for elderly patients.

INTRODUCTION

The global population of individuals aged 65 and above is expected to rise dramatically, increasing from 703 million in 2019 to 1.5 billion by 2050. This growth is primarily driven by advancements in medical science, improved management of health risks, and enhancements in healthcare systems. As a result, the number of older adults facing various health challenges is growing, with many managing multiple chronic conditions that often necessitate polypharmacy. In both developed and developing nations, older individuals frequently use potentially inappropriate medications (PIMs), which can pose risks that may surpass their benefits. Research conducted in India revealed that elderly patients are four times more likely to experience fatal outcomes due to adverse drug reactions (ADRs) compared to children.

The challenge of prescribing medications for older adults stems from several age-related factors, including physiological changes that influence drug pharmacodynamics and pharmacokinetics. Older patients often suffer from multiple chronic and degenerative conditions, leading to an increased number of prescribed medications, which complicates proper medication management. Additionally, there is limited comprehensive data on medication use in older populations, as pharmaceutical companies rarely include older adults in clinical trials before drug approval. Consequently, older individuals are at greater risk of being prescribed PIMs, where the likelihood of adverse effects may surpass the potential benefits.

To address these challenges, healthcare professionals have developed and refined various assessment tools and criteria. These evaluation methods falls into three distinct categories: Explicit criteria based on evidence-based standards, implicit criteria utilizing clinical judgment, and mixed approaches that combine both methodologies **(Table 1)**. The healthcare community has further enhanced these tools through digital integration, creating online platforms that facilitate their practical application in clinical settings.

Table 1 organizes the tools into explicit, implicit, and mixed categories along with their references. It provides a concise and clear overview for clinical or academic use.

The American Geriatrics Society (AGS) Beers Criteria, the Screening Tool of Older People's Potentially Inappropriate Prescriptions (STOPP) criteria, the Screening Tool to Alert Doctors to Right Treatment (START) criteria, the Medication Appropriateness Index (MAI), and the Zhan criteria are key tools that assist healthcare professionals in identifying potentially harmful medications and promoting safer prescribing practices for older adults. In recent years, additional tools have emerged to further address inappropriate prescribing in elderly patients. These include the European Union's list of potentially inappropriate medications [EU(7)-PIM list], Germany's PRISCUS list, and Canada's Improved Prescribing in the Elderly Tool (IPET). These tools serve as valuable resources for healthcare professionals, enhancing medication safety and ensuring appropriate prescribing for elderly populations.

Most experts in geriatric pharmacotherapy agree that regular updates and revisions of explicit criteria for PIMs and potential prescribing omissions (PPOs) are crucial. These updates ensure the criteria remain relevant, incorporate the latest evidence, and enhance medication safety and effectiveness for older adults.

TABLE 1: Assessment tools for polypharmacy.

Type	Tools	Reference/Year
Explicit	Beers Criteria	Fick, Semla, and Steinman, 2019
	Forta Criteria	Kuhn-Thiel, Weiß, and Wehling, 2014
	EU(7)-PIM list	Renom-Guiteras, Meyer, and Thürmann, 2015
	PRISCUS list 2.0	Mann, Mathes, and Sönnichsen, 2023
	STOPP/START Criteria	O'Mahony, Cherubini and Guiteras, 2023
	STOPPFrail Criterion	Lavan, Gallagher, and Parsons, 2017
	TIME-to-STOPP/START Criteria	Bahat, Ilhan, and Erdogan, 2020
	IPET Criteria	Naugler, Brymer, and Stolee, 2000
	NORGEP Criteria	Levy, 2003
	McLeod Criteria	McLeod, Huang, and Tamblyn, 1997
	Rancourt Criteria	Rancourt, Moisan, and Baillargeon, 2004
	Laroche Criteria	Laroche, Charmes, and Merle, 2007
	Online tools (e.g., Fast&Rational web app, TIME Criteria mobile app)	Fast&Rational, 2022
Implicit	Medication Appropriateness Index (MAI)—drug compliance index	Hanlon, Schmader, and Samsa, 1992
	CRIME	Onder, Landi, and Fusco, 2014
	GPGP algorithm	Garfinkel, Zur-Gil, and Ben-Israel, 2007
Mixed	TIMER	Lee, Schwemm, and Reist, 2009
	POM	Drenth-Van Maanen et al.
	ARMOR	Haque, 2009

Source: Adapted from Akyon SH, Silay K, Thurmann PA. Tools to reduce inappropriate drug use in geriatric patients. Arch Gerontol Geriat Plus. 2024;1(4):100052.

BEERS CRITERIA FOR POTENTIALLY INAPPROPRIATE MEDICATIONS

The AGS Beers Criteria® for PIM use in older adults is a widely recognized resource utilized by clinicians, educators, researchers, healthcare administrators, and regulators. Since 2011, the AGS has been responsible for regularly maintaining and updating these criteria. The AGS Beers Criteria® provides a clear list of medications that are generally best avoided in older adults, either in most cases or under specific conditions, such as the presence of certain diseases.

For the 2023 update, an interprofessional expert panel reviewed the most recent evidence published since the 2019 update and approved key changes. These included the addition of new criteria, revisions to existing ones, and formatting improvements to enhance usability. The criteria are designed for adults aged 65 and older across ambulatory, acute, and institutional care settings but exclude hospice and end-of-life care.

Although the AGS Beers Criteria® can be applied internationally, it is specifically tailored to the healthcare context in the United States, with certain medications requiring additional consideration in other countries. Importantly, the criteria are intended to complement, not replace, shared clinical decision-making. The expert panel has categorized the criteria into five general groups:

1. Medications considered as potentially inappropriate
2. Medications potentially inappropriate in patients with certain diseases or syndromes
3. Medications to be used with caution
4. Potentially inappropriate drug-drug interactions
5. Medications whose dosages should be adjusted based on renal function

STOPP/START CRITERIA FOR ELDERLY PATIENTS

The evolution of medication management tools for older adults has been marked by significant developments, with the STOPP/START criteria emerging as a comprehensive approach since their initial introduction in 2008. These criteria serve dual purposes: Identifying medications that should be discontinued (STOPP) and highlighting beneficial treatments that may have been overlooked (START),

The STOPP component organizes PIMs according to physiological systems, aligning with standard drug formulary structures. It includes specialized categories addressing specific risk factors, such as fall risk, opioid use, and anticholinergic burden. Complementing this, the START criteria focus on identifying instances of potential undertreatment, where clinically indicated medications may have been inadvertently omitted from a patient's regimen.

The latest iteration (version 3) represents a substantial expansion of both components. The STOPP criteria have grown from 80 to 133 items (66.25% increase), while the START criteria have expanded from 34 to 57 items (67.6% increase). This expansion reflects the incorporation of new evidence published between 2014 and 2022, particularly regarding the treatment of common age-related conditions such as cardiovascular disease, diabetes, and chronic obstructive pulmonary disease (COPD).

Research has demonstrated the practical benefits of implementing these criteria. A meta-analysis encompassing four randomized controlled trials revealed that utilizing STOPP criteria contributed to reduced instances of falls and delirium among elderly patients. However, the expanding scope of these criteria presents implementation challenges in routine clinical practice. To address this, healthcare providers are increasingly turning to electronic applications that facilitate efficient application of these comprehensive guidelines.

A notable implementation study conducted at a South Indian hospital evaluated prescribing patterns using both Beers 2015 and STOPP criteria. The findings highlighted the potential of these tools to reduce adverse medication events, minimize unnecessary hospitalizations, and optimize healthcare costs in geriatric care. While these criteria provide valuable guidance, they are designed to complement rather than replace clinical judgment.

MEDICATION APPROPRIATENESS INDEX

The MAI represents a distinct approach to medication evaluation, developed in the early 1990s. Unlike criterion-based tools, the MAI employs an implicit methodology that relies on clinical judgment to assess medication appropriateness. This tool utilizes a comprehensive 10-item questionnaire that evaluates medications across multiple domains, including therapeutic indication, effectiveness, dosage optimization, and practical considerations.

The MAI's unique contribution lies in its attention to aspects often overlooked by other tools, such as therapeutic effectiveness, medication administration instructions, and cost considerations. This contrasts with tools like the AGS Beers Criteria and STOPP, which primarily focus on safety considerations and potential contraindications.

Comparative research has demonstrated the MAI's robust capability in identifying potentially inappropriate prescriptions. In a comprehensive study examining 2,645 medications, the MAI identified inappropriate prescribing in 74% of cases, compared to detection rates of 53.1%, 55.7%, and 44.3% for the Beers, STOPP, and FORTA criteria, respectively. The study revealed a particularly strong correlation between polypharmacy (five or more medications) and increased prevalence of potentially inappropriate prescriptions across all evaluation methods.

A separate investigation involving 593 community-dwelling elderly individuals with multiple chronic conditions yielded similar findings. The MAI demonstrated the highest sensitivity, identifying potentially inappropriate prescriptions in 94% of cases, compared to 68.8% and 57.7% for the Beers and STOPP criteria, respectively. The study also revealed that each additional medication corresponded to a 2.41-point increase in the MAI score.

Table 2 simplifies the questions and ratings for evaluating medication appropriateness, aligning with the structure of the MAI.

TABLE 2: Questions and ratings for evaluating medication appropriateness.

Question	Options for rating
1. Is there an indication for the drug?	Indicated/Not indicated
2. Is the medication effective for the condition?	Effective/Ineffective
3. Is the dosage correct?	Correct/Incorrect
4. Are the directions correct?	Correct/Incorrect
5. Are the directions practical?	Practical/Impractical
6. Are there clinically significant drug interactions?	Insignificant/Significant
7. Are there clinically significant drug-disease/condition interactions?	Insignificant/Significant
8. Is there unnecessary duplication with other drug(s)?	Necessary/Unnecessary
9. Is the duration of therapy acceptable?	Acceptable/Not acceptable
10. Is this drug the least expensive alternative compared to others of equal utility?	Least expensive/Most expensive

Source: Adapted from Hanlon JT, Schmader KE. The Medication Appropriateness Index: A Clinimetric Measure. Psychother Psychosom. 2022;91:78-83.

OTHER SCREENING TOOLS FOR OLDER ADULTS

The landscape of medication screening tools continues to evolve with various region-specific and specialized criteria. The Zhan criteria, which adapts elements from the Beers Criteria, provides a streamlined approach by categorizing 33 medications into three distinct groups based on their appropriateness for elderly patients, offering practical guidance for medication safety.

The FORTA (Fit fOR The Aged) system, first implemented in 2008, has undergone significant international adaptation. Through collaborative efforts across seven European nations in 2012, this tool evolved to classify medications for elderly patients with chronic conditions into four systematic categories:

1. Medications demonstrating optimal utility and safety
2. Drugs with established efficacy but potential safety considerations
3. Medications with questionable efficacy and safety profiles
4. Medications to avoid, with recommendations for alternatives

The FORTA framework has seen continuous refinement, with specialized versions emerging to address regional healthcare needs, including EURO-FORTA, US-FORTA, and JAPAN-FORTA in subsequent updates through 2023.

The development of the EU(7)-PIM list in 2015 represented a significant effort to harmonize medication safety standards across Europe. This comprehensive tool synthesized insights from multiple existing criteria, including the PRISCUS 1.0 list, Beers Criteria, Laroche, McLeod, Finnish criteria, and STOPP/START guidelines. Through collaborative expert review across seven European nations, this initiative established a standardized approach to medication safety for elderly patients throughout Europe.

Germany's contribution to medication safety tools began with the PRISCUS 1.0 List in 2010, identifying 83 PIMs across 18 drug categories. The 2023 update to PRISCUS 2.0 marked a substantial expansion, more than doubling its scope to include 177 drug agents, providing healthcare practitioners with more comprehensive guidance for geriatric prescribing.

APPLICATION OF TOOLS IN CLINICAL PRACTICE

Recent research into clinical implementation challenges reveals important insights about tool utilization. A 2022 survey of family medicine residents highlighted two primary obstacles: Difficulty accessing relevant resources and challenges in synthesizing multiple information sources for patient-specific decisions. These findings emphasize the need for integrated digital solutions that provide streamlined access to current guidelines and criteria.

Contemporary digital solutions, such as *TIME and CRITERIA* applications, have emerged to facilitate access to explicit screening criteria. However, the varying scope and limitations of existing tools underscore the need for more comprehensive, updated, and systemically integrated solutions for routine clinical practice.

The *"Fast&Rational"* web platform represents an innovative approach to addressing these challenges. By incorporating six major PIM criteria [EU(7)-PIM, AGS Beers 2019, US-FORTA, Time-to STOPP, STOPP v2, and Priscus 1.0], this tool employs rule-based artificial intelligence to evaluate medication appropriateness. The platform analyzes patient-specific factors including age, current medications, and chronic conditions, generating alerts for potential inappropriate prescribing while providing evidence-based recommendations supported by bibliographic references.

PERCEPTIONS OF INDIAN PHYSICIANS TOWARD DEPRESCRIBING OF MEDICATIONS FOR CHRONIC DISEASES IN ELDERLY

India's demographic transition presents unique challenges in geriatric care. Projections indicate an increase in the elderly population (aged 60 and above) from 7.5% in 2010 to 11.1% by 2025, with southern states expected to experience the most significant demographic shift. National data reveals concerning trends in medication management, with an overall polypharmacy rate of 49% between 2002 and 2020, reaching 65% in northern regions. Additionally, approximately 45% of elderly Indians receive at least one PIM.

A targeted study of 75 physicians revealed important insights into deprescribing practices. The findings showed widespread recognition (92%) of deprescribing benefits, though implementation varied significantly. While 45.3% of physicians reported utilizing the AGS Beers Criteria, only half supported deprescribing certain medication classes, including benzodiazepines, antipsychotics, and antidepressants. Notable barriers to deprescribing included prescriptions from multiple providers (cited by 55% of physicians) and socioeconomic factors (74.6% of respondents).

The limited research on physician perspectives regarding deprescribing in India highlights a critical knowledge gap. As India's elderly population grows rapidly, incorporating standardized assessment tools and criteria into routine clinical practice becomes increasingly important for minimizing adverse events, improving treatment adherence, and enhancing overall clinical outcomes.

CONCLUSION

An individualized approach is essential when determining whether to initiate, discontinue, adjust, or maintain drug therapy in elderly patients. Since certain medications may take years to provide benefits, they may not be appropriate for patients with limited life expectancy and may need to be discontinued. Physicians must not only follow guidelines and criteria but also consider the patient's unique needs, life expectancy, and the anticipated duration of benefit from the medication.

When assessing a patient's medications, it is vital to account for their current health conditions, existing medications, and other key factors such as blood pressure, weight, estimated glomerular filtration rate (eGFR), and glycated hemoglobin (HbA1c). Both explicit and implicit tools for medication evaluation offer distinct advantages and limitations. To address the inconsistencies and shortcomings of current criteria for identifying PIMs, advanced, comprehensive, and user-friendly methods are required for implementation in clinical practice **(Box 1)**.

BOX 1 Recommendation: Criteria and tools for rational prescribing.

Key recommendations for rational prescribing in the elderly

- *Adopt comprehensive prescribing tools*:
  - Use explicit tools such as American Geriatrics Society (AGS) Beers Criteria, STOPP/START Criteria, and FORTA system for evidence-based guidance
  - Incorporate implicit tools such as the Medication Appropriateness Index (MAI) for clinical judgment-based evaluation
  - Leverage mixed tools such as ARMOR and TIMER for a balanced approach to evaluating medication appropriateness
- *Integrate technology for efficiency*:
  - Utilize digital solutions like the Fast&Rational web app or TIME Criteria Mobile App for streamlined application of prescribing tools
  - Implement Clinical Decision Support Systems (CDSS) to enhance medication safety and reduce prescribing errors
- *Regularly update prescribing criteria*:
  - Ensure criteria used are up-to-date with the latest clinical evidence, as seen with tools such as Beers Criteria 2023 and STOPP/START criteria version 3
- *Prioritize patient-centered care*:
  - Engage in shared decision-making, considering patient preferences, health status, and life expectancy
  - Focus on individualized treatment plans tailored to the patient's current medical conditions and therapeutic goals
- *Enhance geriatric training for physicians*:
  - Include training on the use of prescribing tools and deprescribing practices in medical education
  - Emphasize the importance of recognizing potentially inappropriate medications (PIMs) and optimizing medication regimens for elderly patients
- *Promote deprescribing practices*:
  - Regularly evaluate the necessity of medications to minimize polypharmacy and reduce PIMs
  - Address barriers to deprescribing, including prescriptions from multiple providers and patient resistance
- *Monitor and evaluate prescribing practices*:
  - Conduct medication reviews during every patient encounter to assess appropriateness and adherence
  - Use tools like the ARMOR process to assess, review, minimize, optimize, and reassess drug regimens
- *Encourage research and feedback*:
  - Develop region specific tools and guidelines that address local healthcare challenges and demographic needs
  - Facilitate studies to assess the effectiveness of various tools in improving prescribing outcomes

SUGGESTED READINGS

1. Nigussie S, Demeke F. Potentially Inappropriate Medications Use and Associated Factors Among Older Patients on Follow-Up at the Chronic Care Clinic of Hiwot Fana Comprehensive Specialized Hospital in Eastern Ethiopia. Curr Ther Res Clin Exp. 2023;100:100730.
2. McKearney K. Prescribing medicines for elderly patient. Medicine. 2020;48(7):463-7.
3. Fadare JO, Obimakinde AM, Enwere OO, Desalu OO, Ibidapo RO. Physician's Knowledge of Appropriate Prescribing for the Elderly—A Survey Among Family and Internal Medicine Physicians in Nigeria. Front Pharmacol. 2019;10:592.
4. O'Mahony D, Cherubini A, Guiteras AR, Denkinger M, Beuscart JB, Onder G, et al. STOPP/START criteria for potentially inappropriate prescribing in older people: version 3. Eur Geriatr Med. 2023;14:625-32.
5. American Geriatrics Society Beers Criteria® Update Expert Panel. American Geriatrics Society 2023 updated AGS Beers Criteria® for potentially inappropriate medication use in older adults. J Am Geriatr Soc. 2023;71(7):2052-81.
6. ValueinHealth. (2020). PIH75 assessment of the rationality of prescribing in elderly inpatients of a South Indian hospital using Beers 2015 and STOPP criteria. [online] Available from https://www.valueinhealthjournal.com/article/S1098-3015(20)30657-4/fulltext [Last accessed, January, 2025].
7. Hanlon JT, Schmader KE. The Medication Appropriateness Index: A Clinimetric Measure. Psychother Psychosom. 2022;91:78-83.
8. Akyon SH, Sılay K, Thürmann PA. Tools to reduce inappropriate drug use in geriatric patients: PRISCUS 2.0 list updates. Arch Gerontol Geriatr. 2024;1(4):100052.
9. Jawahar S, Selvaraj L, Muruganantham K, Kumar I, Nagasubramanian VR. Perceptions of Indian Physicians towards Deprescribing of Medications for Chronic Diseases in Elderly: A Questionnaire-based Study. Ind J Pharm Edu Res. 2023;57(1s):s160-66.

6

CHAPTER

Personalized Medication Management in Geriatrics

ABSTRACT

The global aging population poses significant challenges for geriatric care, particularly in managing complex medication regimens. Personalized medication management, rooted in the principles of precision medicine, offers an innovative approach to address the unique health needs of older adults. This chapter explores individualized therapeutic strategies that integrate genetic predispositions, comorbidities, drug history, and functional and cognitive status, ensuring safer and more effective pharmacotherapy.

A key focus is placed on the emerging role of pharmacogenomics in managing polypharmacy, where genetic insights into drug metabolism, transport, and response can significantly reduce adverse drug reactions (ADRs) and enhance therapeutic outcomes. Case studies illustrate its application in preventing falls, addressing drug-induced cognitive impairment, and managing chronic pain and inflammation. For instance, identifying genetic variations in enzymes such as CYP2D6 and CYP2C9 informs tailored dosing and drug selection, improving safety and efficacy in high-risk patients.

The chapter also underscores the indispensable role of caregivers in supporting adherence, monitoring for side effects, and bridging communication gaps with healthcare providers. Caregivers' involvement, combined with shared decision-making, fosters collaboration between patients, families, and clinicians, aligning therapeutic goals with individual preferences and enhancing patient satisfaction. By integrating regular monitoring, pharmacogenomic insights, and evidence-based deprescribing strategies, this chapter highlights the transformative potential of personalized medication management in achieving safe, effective, and patient-centered care for elderly populations.

INTRODUCTION

The global aging population has led to an unprecedented increase in the demand for specialized geriatric care, with an emphasis on addressing the unique health challenges faced by older adults. This demographic shift brings about complexities in medical management, as older adults are often affected by multiple chronic conditions requiring intricate pharmacological regimens. The confluence of these conditions, coupled with age-related physiological changes, amplifies the risk of adverse drug reactions (ADRs), drug-drug interactions, and overall medication burden. Consequently, a focused and systematic approach to geriatric medicine has become indispensable.

PRECISION MEDICINE IN GERIATRIC CARE

Precision medicine represents a paradigm shift in healthcare, moving beyond the traditional "one-size-fits-all" approach to treatment. In geriatric populations, precision medicine emphasizes individualized therapeutic strategies by integrating a wide range of patient-specific factors, including:

- *Genetic predispositions:* Variations in pharmacogenomics affect how drugs are metabolized and can guide safer and more effective prescribing practices.
- *Comorbidities:* The presence of multiple chronic diseases often necessitates careful prioritization of therapies to avoid drug-disease interactions.
- *Drug history and adherence patterns:* A history of prior medication use informs the risks of cumulative side effects or ADRs.
- *Social and demographic factors:* Socioeconomic status, support systems, and access to healthcare services influence medication adherence and outcomes.

Precision medicine acknowledges the biological, clinical, and social heterogeneity among older adults, recognizing that these factors collectively impact the efficacy and safety of therapeutic interventions. By leveraging data-driven insights, clinicians can tailor interventions to meet the specific needs of each patient, enhancing both outcomes and quality of life.

CHALLENGES IN GERIATRIC PHARMACOTHERAPY

The complexity of medication management in older adults stems from several intrinsic challenges:

- *Polypharmacy:* Defined as the concurrent use of five or more medications, polypharmacy increases the likelihood of ADRs and drug interactions. Studies indicate a strong association between polypharmacy and conditions such as cognitive decline, falls, and hospitalizations.
- *Physiological changes with aging:* Reduced renal and hepatic function alters drug clearance, necessitating dosage adjustments to prevent toxicity.
- *Cognitive and functional impairments:* These may hinder adherence to prescribed regimens, complicating therapeutic goals.
- *Economic constraints:* Limited financial resources may lead to prioritization of medications, often at the cost of adherence or optimal therapy.

TOWARDS INDIVIDUALIZED AND MULTIDISCIPLINARY MANAGEMENT

In response to these complexities, geriatricians must adopt a multidisciplinary and patient-centered approach to medication management. Individualized care, guided by comprehensive assessments of each patient's clinical and functional status, forms the foundation of effective geriatric pharmacotherapy.

The integration of shared decision-making (SDM) and deprescribing frameworks ensures that treatment plans align with patient goals and minimize unnecessary medication burdens.

This chapter explores the critical aspects of personalized medication management in geriatrics, including:

- Strategies for adapting drug therapy to patient-specific factors
- The importance of dosage adjustments in mitigating the risks of ADRs
- The role of caregivers and families in supporting adherence and monitoring
- The application of deprescribing techniques to reduce polypharmacy

By highlighting these facets, the chapter aims to provide healthcare practitioners with actionable insights and evidence-based strategies to optimize pharmacological care for older adults, ensuring safety, efficacy, and sustainability in medication management.

INDIVIDUALIZED DRUG THERAPY BASED ON PATIENT-SPECIFIC FACTORS

The effectiveness and safety of pharmacotherapy in elderly populations are heavily influenced by individual patient factors. Older adults often have complex clinical profiles due to multiple chronic conditions, varied medication histories, and differences in functional and cognitive status. Individualizing drug therapy is paramount to address these unique needs, ensuring optimal therapeutic outcomes and minimizing the risk of ADRs.

Comorbidities

Older adults commonly present with multiple chronic diseases, a phenomenon that necessitates polypharmacy—often leading to drug-disease and drug-drug interactions. Proper management of comorbidities requires a nuanced approach to prioritize treatments while minimizing potential risks.

Drug-disease interactions: Tailoring pharmacotherapy involves a comprehensive understanding of how medications interact with preexisting conditions. For instance:

- *Nonsteroidal anti-inflammatory drugs (NSAIDs):* These can exacerbate kidney damage in patients with chronic renal insufficiency, making alternative pain management strategies essential.
- *Beta-blockers in chronic obstructive pulmonary disease (COPD) patients:* These may worsen respiratory symptoms, requiring careful consideration of alternative options.

Prioritization of treatments: The *STOPP/START criteria* (Screening Tool of Older People's Prescriptions and Screening Tool to Alert Doctors to the Right Treatment) provide a robust framework to identify and address potentially inappropriate medications (PIMs). This includes deprescribing medications that no longer provide benefit while ensuring that gaps in therapy are filled. For example:

- *Benzodiazepines* are discouraged in elderly patients due to their association with falls and cognitive impairment, especially when safer alternatives such as nonpharmacological interventions for anxiety or insomnia are available.

Drug History

A detailed review of a patient's drug history is a cornerstone of individualized therapy. This process involves analyzing past medication use to identify patterns of tolerance, adherence, and previous ADRs.

Historical insights: Understanding prior medication use helps identify drugs that were previously effective or caused complications. For example:

- A history of statin-induced myopathy can guide the selection of alternative lipid-lowering therapies.
- Cases of antibiotic misuse leading to complications like resistance or ADRs emphasize the need for evidence-based prescribing.

Tools for Medication Reconciliation

Comprehensive medication reviews (CMRs): These involve evaluating all prescribed, over-the-counter, and herbal medications to avoid duplication and interactions.

Effective medication reviews ensure that therapies remain aligned with a patient's current clinical needs while mitigating unnecessary risks.

Functional and Cognitive Status

Functional and cognitive impairments significantly influence the appropriateness of drug regimens in elderly patients. These factors necessitate adjustments in medication types, dosing schedules, and delivery methods.

Cognitive Impairment

- *Anticholinergics and sedatives* are known to exacerbate cognitive decline and frailty in older adults. Such medications should be avoided or used with caution.
- Tools like the *Anticholinergic Burden Scale* provide a quantitative measure of a patient's exposure to these drugs, guiding safer prescribing practices.

Functional Considerations

- Simplified regimens (e.g., combination therapies or once-daily dosing) improve adherence, especially in patients with mobility or dexterity issues.
- Aligning medication plans with a patient's physical capabilities ensures that therapies remain practical and achievable.

Addressing functional and cognitive needs not only reduces ADR risks but also improves quality of life and treatment adherence.

DOSAGE ADJUSTMENT IN THE ELDERLY

Aging induces physiological changes that affect drug pharmacokinetics and pharmacodynamics, requiring precise dose adjustments to optimize efficacy while minimizing toxicity.

Pharmacokinetics

- *Absorption:* While drug absorption is often unaffected, slower gastric emptying can delay drug onset in elderly patients.

- *Distribution:* Increased fat mass and reduced lean body mass alter the distribution of lipophilic drugs such as benzodiazepines, prolonging their half-life and effects.
- *Metabolism:* Reduced hepatic enzyme activity affects the metabolism of drugs such as benzodiazepines and opioids, necessitating lower starting doses.
- *Excretion:* Declined renal function with age reduces drug clearance, especially for renally excreted drugs such as aminoglycosides and digoxin, increasing the risk of accumulation and toxicity.

Guidelines for Dosing

- The *Beers Criteria* and renal dosing calculators provide evidence-based recommendations for dose modifications in older adults, ensuring that pharmacokinetics is appropriately considered.
- *Example:* Dosage adjustments for renally cleared drugs such as metformin and aminoglycosides prevent the risk of lactic acidosis and nephrotoxicity, respectively.

Individualized drug therapy in geriatrics requires a holistic approach that incorporates comorbidities, drug history, and functional and cognitive status. Dose adjustments informed by pharmacokinetic changes are essential to prevent ADRs and optimize therapeutic outcomes. By leveraging tools such as CMRs, the STOPP/START criteria, and dosing guidelines, clinicians can deliver safer and more effective care tailored to the unique needs of older adults.

Monitoring and Reviewing Drug Therapy Regularly

Effective medication management for older adults hinges on continuous monitoring and regular review of drug therapy. This process ensures that the prescribed treatments remain appropriate as patients' clinical and functional statuses evolve. Regular monitoring helps clinicians achieve therapeutic goals, minimize ADRs, and adapt regimens in response to changes in patient needs or conditions. One of the most effective frameworks for achieving these objectives is *clinical pharmacological reconciliation, review, and feedback (CPRRF).*

The Role of Clinical Pharmacological Reconciliation, Review, and Feedback in Geriatric Pharmacotherapy

Clinical pharmacological reconciliation, review, and feedback is a structured methodology designed to optimize medication use and enhance patient safety in geriatric populations. This framework involves three interconnected components.

Medication Reconciliation at Transitions of Care

Transitions of care, such as hospital admissions, discharges, or shifts between primary and specialty care, are critical points where medication errors are most likely to occur.

Medication reconciliation is the process of verifying and updating a patient's complete medication list at these junctures. It involves identifying discrepancies, such as duplicate therapies, omissions, or incorrect dosages.

Example: An elderly patient transitioning from hospital to home care was found to have multiple duplicate prescriptions for antihypertensives. Through reconciliation, the regimen was streamlined, reducing the risk of hypotension and falls.

Proactive Adverse Drug Reaction Management through Interdisciplinary Collaboration

Adverse drug reactions are a leading cause of morbidity among older adults. Effective ADR management requires collaboration among healthcare providers, including physicians, pharmacists, and nurses.

Interdisciplinary teams proactively monitor for ADRs using tools such as the Beers Criteria and Anticholinergic Burden Scale to identify high-risk medications.

Example: In a geriatric outpatient clinic, routine collaboration between a clinical pharmacist and the primary care physician led to the early identification of gastrointestinal bleeding caused by NSAID use, prompting a switch to safer alternatives.

Leveraging Technology for Real-time Monitoring

Electronic health records (EHRs): EHRs enable real-time tracking of medication regimens, alerting clinicians to potential drug-drug interactions, missed doses, or adherence issues.

Clinical decision support systems (CDSS): Integrated into EHRs, CDSS can flag high-risk prescriptions based on patient-specific factors, such as renal impairment or known allergies.

Example: A case study demonstrated that EHR-integrated alerts helped prevent prescribing a contraindicated statin to a patient with liver disease.

CASE STUDIES ILLUSTRATING THE EFFICACY OF CLINICAL PHARMACOLOGICAL RECONCILIATION, REVIEW, AND FEEDBACK

The CPRRF methodology has demonstrated substantial benefits in optimizing drug therapy and improving patient outcomes in geriatric populations. The following detailed case studies illustrate its impact in reducing polypharmacy, addressing ADR cascades, and optimizing transitions of care.

Reducing Polypharmacy through Deprescribing

Case details: An 80-year-old female patient was prescribed 12 medications to manage chronic conditions, including diabetes, hypertension, and osteoarthritis. Despite adherence, she experienced persistent fatigue, confusion, and daytime somnolence, which significantly impacted her quality of life. Her caregiver reported difficulties in managing the medication regimen, leading to frequent dosing errors.

Clinical Pharmacological Reconciliation, Review, and Feedback Evaluation

Medication Reconciliation

The review identified redundant medications, including two antihypertensives with overlapping mechanisms and an over-the-counter sleep aid contributing to her cognitive impairment.

High anticholinergic burden was noted from medications prescribed for osteoarthritis pain and insomnia.

Interdisciplinary Collaboration

A clinical pharmacologist flagged medications with potential interactions and ADRs, such as a combination of anticholinergics and sedatives.

Recommendations were discussed with the primary care physician, focusing on deprescribing non-essential medications.

Outcome

Four medications were deprescribed, including a sleep aid and one antihypertensive, reducing the total regimen to eight medications.

The patient reported significant improvements in cognitive function, increased alertness, and decreased fatigue within 4 weeks.

Follow-up visits confirmed better medication adherence, as the simplified regimen was easier for both the patient and caregiver to manage.

This case underscores the efficacy of CPRRF in addressing polypharmacy, streamlining drug regimens, and improving geriatric patients' cognitive and functional outcomes.

PREVENTING ADVERSE DRUG REACTION CASCADES

Case details: A 67-year-old female with a history of urinary incontinence was prescribed an anticholinergic medication. She subsequently developed severe dry mouth and dizziness, symptoms which were misinterpreted as new conditions. To address these issues, additional medications, including a saliva stimulant and a low-dose benzodiazepine, were prescribed. This cascade of prescriptions led to worsening cognitive impairment and falls.

Clinical Pharmacological Reconciliation, Review, and Feedback Evaluation

Medication Review

The anticholinergic medication was identified as the root cause of her dry mouth and dizziness.

Additional prescribed medications were deemed unnecessary and contributing to further adverse outcomes.

Feedback and Adjustment

The anticholinergic medication was discontinued, and alternative non-pharmacological interventions for urinary incontinence were suggested.

A comprehensive plan was created to manage the patient's condition without initiating new medications.

Outcome

Within 2 weeks, the patient's dry mouth and dizziness resolved completely.

Discontinuation of the benzodiazepine improved her alertness and reduced her risk of falls.

The patient and her family expressed relief over the simplified treatment plan and its effectiveness.

This case highlights how CPRRF can interrupt prescribing cascades, prevent ADRs, and emphasize the importance of addressing the underlying causes of symptoms rather than layering medications.

OPTIMIZING TRANSITIONS OF CARE

Case details: A 75-year-old male with congestive heart failure (CHF) was discharged from the hospital with a new prescription for diuretics to manage fluid retention. At home, the patient developed severe dehydration and electrolyte imbalances, resulting in confusion, muscle cramps, and weakness. A post-discharge review revealed that he was taking the diuretics at incorrect doses due to poorly communicated instructions.

Clinical Pharmacological Reconciliation, Review, and Feedback Evaluation

Medication Reconciliation

A thorough review of the patient's medications identified that the diuretic dose was significantly higher than recommended for his renal function.

Lack of a clear titration plan at discharge contributed to the overdose.

Interdisciplinary Coordination

A heart failure specialist and pharmacist collaborated to reassess the patient's treatment regimen.

Adjustments were made to reduce the diuretic dose and include electrolyte supplementation.

Feedback and Education

Clear, written instructions were provided to the patient and his caregiver, emphasizing the correct timing and dosage of medications.

Regular follow-ups were scheduled to monitor electrolyte levels and fluid status.

Outcome

Symptoms of dehydration resolved within 1 week, and the patient's electrolyte levels normalized.

Subsequent follow-ups showed improved adherence and understanding of the medication plan.

The patient's CHF symptoms were effectively managed without further complications.

Conclusion

This case demonstrates the importance of CPRRF in ensuring safe transitions of care, reducing the risk of post-discharge complications, and promoting effective communication between healthcare providers and patients.

SUMMARY OF IMPACT

These case studies exemplify the transformative potential of CPRRF in geriatric pharmacotherapy. Key outcomes include:

- Enhanced safety through deprescribing and ADR prevention.
- Improved quality of life by addressing medication-related cognitive and functional impairments.
- Streamlined care transitions, reducing medication errors, and complications.
- By employing CPRRF methodologies, healthcare teams can achieve sustainable improvements in drug therapy management, making a significant difference in the lives of older adults and their caregivers.

BENEFITS OF REGULAR MONITORING AND CLINICAL PHARMACOLOGICAL RECONCILIATION, REVIEW, AND FEEDBACK IMPLEMENTATION

- *Enhanced patient safety:* By identifying and mitigating risks early, CPRRF reduces hospitalizations and emergency visits.
- *Improved therapeutic outcomes:* Regular monitoring ensures that medications are aligned with the patient's current health status and therapeutic goals.
- *Cost-effective care:* Streamlining regimens through deprescribing eliminates unnecessary medications, reducing healthcare costs for patients and systems alike.
- *Patient-centered approach:* Ongoing reviews involve patients and caregivers in discussions about their medications, fostering SDM and adherence.

Regular monitoring and the adoption of CPRRF principles are essential components of personalized geriatric care. By combining meticulous reconciliation, interdisciplinary collaboration, and advanced technology, clinicians can ensure that drug therapy remains safe, effective, and tailored to the needs of older adults. This approach not only enhances the quality of care but also empowers patients to achieve better health outcomes.

SHARED DECISION-MAKING IN MEDICATION PRESCRIBING

Shared decision-making is a collaborative process that actively involves patients in their treatment decisions, fostering adherence, satisfaction, and better health outcomes. Unlike the traditional paternalistic approach, which places decision-making solely in the hands of healthcare providers, SDM emphasizes a partnership between clinicians, patients, and their families. This approach is particularly critical in geriatric care, where treatment plans must align with the patient's preferences, functional status, and lifestyle goals.

Key Components of Shared Decision-making

Educational Approaches: Simplifying Benefits and Risks

Patients often find medical information overwhelming, particularly when dealing with complex medication regimens. Effective SDM requires simplifying technical jargon into accessible language, helping patients understand:

- *The benefits of treatment:* How the prescribed medication will improve their symptoms, quality of life, or long-term outcomes.
- *The risks involved:* Potential adverse effects, interactions, and how to recognize early signs of complications.

Tools to Enhance Understanding

- Visual aids, such as diagrams or charts, can effectively explain treatment effects.
- Decision aids, including pamphlets or digital tools, can outline options and associated risks to support informed choices.

Example: A patient prescribed anticoagulants for atrial fibrillation might receive simplified information comparing the risks of bleeding with the benefits of stroke prevention, empowering them to weigh their options.

Collaborative Goal Setting: Aligning Therapy with Patient Goals

- Geriatric patients often prioritize quality of life over aggressive treatments that might lead to significant side effects or require burdensome regimens.
- Collaborative goal setting involves discussing and aligning the treatment plan with the patient's values, such as:
  - Maintaining independence and mobility
  - Minimizing the burden of polypharmacy
  - Reducing medication costs if financial constraints are present.

Example: A patient with mild dementia might prioritize maintaining cognitive clarity, leading the care team to avoid medications with high anticholinergic burdens, even if they are indicated for other conditions.

Challenges in Practice: Overcoming Barriers

Literacy and Health Literacy

- Low health literacy levels in some populations can make it difficult for patients to understand medication instructions or risks.
- Strategies to overcome these barriers include using simple language, avoiding medical jargon, and providing information in multiple formats (e.g., verbal, written, or video).

Cultural Sensitivity

- Cultural norms may influence how patients perceive healthcare and decision-making authority. In some cultures, patients may defer entirely to their physician or involve family members extensively in decisions.
- Healthcare providers must adapt their communication style to honor these cultural preferences while still encouraging patient participation.

Cognitive Impairments

Patients with cognitive decline may struggle to engage in SDM fully. In such cases, involving caregivers or family members ensures that decisions are made in the patient's best interest.

The Transformative Potential of Shared Decision-making

Shared decision-making transforms the prescriptive approach into a dynamic partnership, empowering patients and families to take an active role in healthcare. The key benefits include:

- *Increased adherence:* When patients understand and agree with the rationale for their treatment, they are more likely to adhere to the regimen.
- *Enhanced satisfaction:* Patients feel respected and valued when their preferences and concerns are acknowledged, leading to higher satisfaction with their care.
- *Improved outcomes:* Aligning treatment with a patient's goals reduces the likelihood of conflicts or non-adherence, ultimately leading to better clinical and quality-of-life outcomes.

Practical Implementation of Shared Decision-making

To embed SDM into routine practice, clinicians can adopt the following steps:

- *Initiate the discussion*: Encourage open communication by asking patients about their goals, concerns, and expectations regarding their treatment.
- *Present options*: Outline all viable treatment options, including their risks, benefits, and potential outcomes, using patient-friendly materials.
- *Facilitate deliberation*: Allow patients time to consider their options, discuss them with their family, and ask questions.
- *Make a joint decision*: Collaboratively agree on a treatment plan that aligns with the patient's preferences and clinical needs.
- *Follow-up*: Monitor the patient's progress and reassess their goals and preferences as their health evolves.

Shared decision-making is a cornerstone of patient-centered care in geriatrics, promoting adherence, satisfaction, and better outcomes. By simplifying communication, aligning therapy with patient goals, and addressing barriers such as health literacy and cultural differences, clinicians can build trust and empower patients to take an active role in their healthcare. This collaborative model not only enhances the quality of care but also ensures that treatment plans resonate with what matters most to the patient.

ROLE OF CAREGIVERS AND FAMILY MEMBERS IN MEDICATION MANAGEMENT

Caregivers and family members are indispensable in the management of medications for older adults, particularly those with chronic conditions, cognitive impairments, or physical limitations. Their involvement bridges the gap between the patient and healthcare providers, ensuring continuity of care and adherence to prescribed regimens. Caregivers not only provide practical support but also act as advocates and monitors for potential issues like ADRs. Their role can significantly influence the success of therapeutic outcomes and the overall quality of life for the patient.

KEY ROLES AND RESPONSIBILITIES OF CAREGIVERS IN MEDICATION MANAGEMENT

Practical Support

Organizing medications: Caregivers often take on the responsibility of sorting and preparing medications to simplify administration. Tools such as pill organizers, labeled storage containers, and digital reminders can help streamline this process.

For patients on polypharmacy regimens, caregivers ensure that medications are taken at the correct times and in the appropriate dosages, reducing the risk of errors.

Maintaining schedules: Medication adherence requires precise timing, particularly for drugs with narrow therapeutic windows or complex regimens. Caregivers monitor and enforce adherence by setting reminders or physically administering the medications.

Observing behavioral and physical changes: Since caregivers are often closest to the patient, they are well-positioned to notice subtle behavioral or physical changes that may indicate ADRs, medication inefficacy, or disease progression.

Example: A caregiver might observe increased confusion or lethargy after starting a new medication, prompting a timely review by the healthcare team.

Communication Bridges

- *Translating healthcare instructions:* Medical advice and instructions can sometimes be overwhelming or unclear for patients, especially if they have low health literacy or cognitive impairments. Caregivers act as intermediaries, simplifying and translating these instructions into actionable steps for the patient.
    - *Example:* A caregiver may create a color-coded chart to explain a complex medication schedule provided by the healthcare provider.
- *Facilitating dialogue with healthcare teams:* Caregivers often accompany patients to medical appointments, where they can relay concerns, report observed side effects and seek clarification on treatment plans.

In multicultural settings, caregivers may help overcome language and cultural barriers, ensuring the patient's needs are effectively communicated and understood.

Training Initiatives

- *Recognizing ADRs and side effects:* Caregivers are often the first to notice side effects or signs of ADRs, such as rash, gastrointestinal discomfort, or behavioral changes. Empowering them to recognize these symptoms ensures early intervention and reduces the risk of complications.

- *Example:* Training caregivers to use tools like the Anticholinergic Burden Scale can help them identify potentially harmful medications contributing to cognitive impairment or frailty.
- *Engaging with healthcare teams:* Caregivers should be equipped to communicate effectively with healthcare providers, whether to report observed issues, inquire about alternative treatments, or discuss deprescribing options.
  - *Example*: A caregiver noticing a decline in mobility after starting a sedative might raise concerns with the provider, prompting a review and possible adjustment of the medication.
- *Educational programs:* Community health programs or workshops can train caregivers in medication management, focusing on topics such as proper storage, safe administration techniques, and recognizing drug interactions.

CHALLENGES FACED BY CAREGIVERS AND STRATEGIES TO OVERCOME THEM

- *Emotional and physical burden:*
  - Managing medications can be stressful and time-consuming, particularly when dealing with complex regimens or uncooperative patients.
  - *Solution:* Respite care and support groups can help caregivers manage their own well-being, preventing burnout.
- *Knowledge gaps*:
  - Many caregivers lack formal training in recognizing ADRs or handling complex medication schedules.
  - *Solution:* Structured educational initiatives, including instructional videos, one-on-one coaching by healthcare providers, and access to online resources, can bridge this gap.
- *Coordination with healthcare providers*:
  - Caregivers may face difficulties accessing or understanding medical records, limiting their ability to contribute effectively.
  - *Solution:* Encourage the use of patient portals or digital health tools that caregivers can access to stay updated on medication changes and clinical instructions.

THE IMPACT OF CAREGIVER INVOLVEMENT

When caregivers are effectively involved in medication management, the benefits are far-reaching:

- *Improved adherence*: Studies show that patients are more likely to adhere to prescribed regimens when caregivers actively oversee medication administration.
- *Reduced risk of adverse drug reactions*: Caregivers' vigilance in observing and reporting side effects ensures timely adjustments to treatment plans.
- *Enhanced patient-centered care*: By incorporating caregivers into the care team, clinicians can tailor treatment plans to align with the patient's lifestyle, preferences, and support system.

- *Empowerment and advocacy*: Caregivers empowered with knowledge and tools become strong advocates for the patient, ensuring that their needs and concerns are addressed promptly.

Caregivers and family members play an essential role in the medication management of older adults, bridging gaps between patients and healthcare providers. By organizing medications, maintaining schedules, and observing for side effects, caregivers provide practical support. Through effective communication and training initiatives, they ensure adherence and enable early detection of potential issues, significantly enhancing the safety and quality of care. Supporting and educating caregivers in these roles not only benefits patients but also strengthens the overall healthcare ecosystem, ensuring holistic and patient-centered treatment.

PHARMACOGENOMICS IN POLYPHARMACY

Pharmacogenomics, the study of how genetic variations affect an individual's response to drugs, has significant implications in the context of polypharmacy, especially in elderly populations. Polypharmacy, defined as the concurrent use of five or more medications, is often necessary due to the high prevalence of multimorbidity among older adults. However, it also increases the risks of drug-drug, drug-disease, and drug-gene interactions, potentially leading to ADRs or suboptimal treatment outcomes.

Pharmacogenomics offers a promising avenue to mitigate these risks by tailoring medication regimens based on the patient's genetic makeup. By integrating genomic insights into clinical decision-making, healthcare providers can optimize drug efficacy, reduce ADRs, and enhance the overall safety of pharmacotherapy in older adults. This section explores the role of pharmacogenomics in addressing the challenges of polypharmacy, particularly in the areas of falls and fractures, cognitive impairment, chronic pain and inflammation, and infectious diseases.

Pharmacogenomics and Falls/Fractures in the Elderly

Falls and fractures are common in older adults and can be both a result of underlying diseases and ADRs. Multiple drug classes, such as sedatives, antidepressants, and antipsychotics, are associated with an increased risk of falls. Nearly 50% of these drugs are substrates for polymorphic drug-metabolizing enzymes such as *CYP2C19* and *CYP2D6*, making genetic variations in these pathways' critical determinants of drug safety and efficacy.

Case Study

An 82-year-old male with Parkinson's disease was prescribed an antipsychotic for agitation. Shortly after initiating treatment, he experienced frequent falls. Pharmacogenomic testing revealed he was a poor metabolizer of CYP2D6 substrates, leading to higher plasma concentrations of the antipsychotic, exacerbating sedation and orthostatic hypotension. Adjusting the dose and switching to a drug with a lower CYP2D6 dependency resolved the issue, reducing his fall risk.

This example illustrates how integrating pharmacogenomics into drug selection and dosing decisions can minimize fall-related risks in elderly patients.

Drug-induced Cognitive Impairment and Genomics

Cognitive impairment is a significant concern in geriatric pharmacotherapy, often resulting from ADRs or complex interactions between drugs and underlying conditions. Two forms of cognitive impairment are observed:

- *Dose-related cognitive impairment:* It is seen with sedatives and other central nervous system (CNS)-active drugs, where nearly all users experience some degree of cognitive decline.
- *Idiosyncratic cognitive impairment:* It occurs in a genetically predisposed subgroup exposed to specific drugs, such as fluoroquinolones or tacrolimus.

Case Study

A 78-year-old female with urinary tract infection was prescribed ciprofloxacin. Within days, she exhibited confusion and hallucinations. Pharmacogenomic analysis identified a variant in the *ABCB1* gene, which encodes a transporter affecting blood-brain barrier permeability. This variant increased CNS exposure to ciprofloxacin, precipitating neurotoxicity. Discontinuing ciprofloxacin and initiating an alternative therapy resolved her symptoms.

Pharmacogenomic insights are particularly valuable in identifying patients at risk for idiosyncratic reactions and guiding safer prescribing.

Chronic Pain, Inflammation, and Genomics

Chronic pain and systemic inflammation significantly impact the quality of life in elderly patients, many of whom rely on NSAIDs. These drugs carry a heightened risk of gastrointestinal (GI) bleeding in older adults, particularly in those treated with anticoagulants or carrying specific genetic variants.

Case Study

A 75-year-old male on NSAIDs for osteoarthritis pain presented with severe GI bleeding. Genetic testing revealed a **CYP2C93/3 genotype, associated with slower metabolism of NSAIDs, leading to higher drug levels and increased bleeding risk. Reducing the NSAID dose and introducing a gastroprotective agent reduced his symptoms and prevented further complications.

Genomic testing can identify patients at heightened risk of ADRs, enabling more precise dosing and the use of alternative therapies to manage pain and inflammation.

Pharmacogenomics in Infectious Diseases

Infectious diseases are a major cause of morbidity and mortality among older adults, often exacerbated by age-related immune dysregulation. Genomic testing offers potential for individualized antibiotic therapy and targeted interventions based on immune function.

Case Study

A 70-year-old female with recurrent pneumonia was treated with broad-spectrum antibiotics, leading to suboptimal outcomes and frequent relapses. Pharmacogenomic testing identified a polymorphism in the *SLCO1B1* gene, affecting the transport of certain antibiotics and reducing their efficacy. Switching to a more effective antibiotic based on her genetic profile resolved her infection and prevented future relapses.

This case underscores the utility of pharmacogenomics in optimizing treatment for infectious diseases in the elderly.

Challenges and Future Directions

Despite its potential, pharmacogenomics in polypharmacy faces challenges:

- *Lack of clinical data:* Randomized controlled trials cannot account for the vast combinations of genetic variations, diseases, and drug regimens in elderly populations.
- *Integration into practice:* Currently, pharmacogenomics is not widely included in deprescribing algorithms or lists of PIMs.
- *Age-related genomic variations:* Emerging research suggests that acquired somatic mutations in the elderly may influence drug response, requiring further exploration.

Future research should focus on identifying actionable biomarkers, improving access to genomic testing, and integrating pharmacogenomic insights into clinical guidelines.

Pharmacogenomics offers a pathway to safer and more effective medication management in elderly patients experiencing polypharmacy. By addressing genetic variations that affect drug metabolism, transport, and response, healthcare providers can individualize therapy to reduce ADRs, improve outcomes, and enhance patient safety. Case studies highlight its relevance in managing complex conditions such as falls, cognitive impairment, chronic pain, and infections. As research advances, pharmacogenomics holds the promise of transforming geriatric pharmacotherapy into a more precise and patient-centered discipline.

CONCLUSION

Personalized medication management in geriatrics is a critical component of improving outcomes for the aging population. This chapter demonstrates how precision medicine, with its emphasis on patient-specific factors, can address the challenges of polypharmacy, ADRs, and complex drug-disease interactions. Strategies such as dosage adjustments based on pharmacokinetics, regular monitoring through frameworks such as CPRRF, and integrating pharmacogenomics into clinical decision-making enhance the safety and efficacy of geriatric pharmacotherapy.

Additionally, SDM fosters collaboration between patients, caregivers, and healthcare providers, aligning therapeutic goals with patient values and lifestyles.

The involvement of caregivers plays a pivotal role in ensuring adherence, monitoring for side effects, and bridging communication gaps with healthcare teams. Pharmacogenomics offers a promising frontier in addressing the genetic underpinnings of drug response, enabling safer and more effective therapies for complex conditions such as falls, cognitive impairment, chronic pain, and infections.

Despite current limitations, including insufficient clinical data and the need for greater integration into practice, the future of geriatric pharmacotherapy lies in advancing precision medicine. By leveraging actionable biomarkers and genomic insights, clinicians can transform medication management into a more precise, patient-centered discipline that prioritizes the quality of life and well-being of older adults **(Box 1)**.

BOX 1 Recommendations—personalized medication management in geriatrics.

- *Individualizing drug therapy*:
  - Use tools such as the STOPP/START criteria and comprehensive medication reviews (CMRs) to identify inappropriate medications
  - Adjust medication regimens based on comorbidities, functional status, and pharmacokinetics (e.g., Beers Criteria for dosage adjustments)
- *Pharmacogenomics in practice*:
  - Integrate pharmacogenomic testing for drugs metabolized by polymorphic enzymes (e.g., CYP2D6, CYP2C9) to minimize adverse drug reactions (ADRs)
  - Prioritize pharmacogenomics in high-risk areas such as:
    - Falls and fractures (e.g., sedatives and antipsychotics)
    - Drug-induced cognitive impairment (e.g., CNS-active medications)
    - Pain management (e.g., NSAIDs with gastroprotective strategies)
- *Monitoring and reviewing medications*:
  - Apply clinical pharmacological reconciliation, review, and feedback (CPRRF):
    - Perform regular medication reconciliations, especially during care transitions
    - Utilize electronic health record (EHR) and clinical decision support systems (CDSS) tools to identify high-risk prescriptions
- *Shared decision-making*:
  - Involve patients and caregivers in all stages of decision-making to align therapeutic goals with patient values
  - Simplify complex regimens with visual aids and written instructions
- *Role of caregivers*:
  - Train caregivers in recognizing ADRs and understanding medication schedules
  - Provide caregivers with access to patient portals and medication tracking tools
- *Deprescribing strategies*:
  - Prioritize deprescribing in cases of polypharmacy, focusing on medications with high anticholinergic burden or low therapeutic benefit
  - Consider the role of pharmacogenomics when evaluating potentially inappropriate drugs

SUGGESTED READINGS

1. Austin CA, Seligman B, Shan-Bala S, Kuchel GA, Loh KP, Kistler CE, et al. Aging precisely: Precision medicine through the lens of an older adult. J Am Geriatr Soc. 2024;72(10):2972-80.
2. Siafarikas N. Personalized medicine in old age psychiatry and Alzheimer's disease. Front Psychiatry. 2024;15:1297798.
3. Samajdar SS, Mukherjee S, Sharma J, Pal J, Tripathi SK, Saboo B, et al. Clinical pharmacological reconciliation, review, and feedback in elderly care: a transformative approach. J Indian Acad Geriatr. 2024;20(3):150-3.
4. Henney AM. The promise and challenge of personalized medicine: aging populations, complex diseases, and unmet medical need. Croat Med J. 2012;53(3):207-10.
5. Samajdar SS, Chatterjee N, Pal J, George M, Sarkar S, Sen S, et al. Rational Deprescribing Practices in Elderly Patients: An Expert Opinion. Bengal Phys J. 2024;11(3):133-45.
6. Božina N, Vrkić Kirhmajer M, Šimičević L, Ganoci L, Mirošević Skvrce N, Klarica Domjanović I, et al. Use of pharmacogenomics in elderly patients treated for cardiovascular diseases. Croat Med J. 2020;61(2):147-58.

7

CHAPTER

Ethical and Legal Considerations in Prescribing for the Elderly

ABSTRACT

Prescribing for elderly patients requires a nuanced approach that balances ethical principles, patient autonomy, and legal responsibilities. This chapter explores key challenges in managing medications for elderly populations, including informed consent, ethical dilemmas, deprescribing practices, and end-of-life care. It emphasizes the importance of shared decision-making, addressing over- and undertreatment, and navigating legal obligations such as documentation, adherence to guidelines, and substituted decision-making. Practical examples illustrate strategies to ensure patient-centered care, uphold ethical standards, and achieve optimal outcomes for elderly patients.

INTRODUCTION

The aging population presents unique challenges in medication management due to age-related physiological changes, chronic conditions, and variable life expectancies. Ethical and legal considerations are integral to prescribing for the elderly, given the potential for cognitive impairments, communication barriers, and complex treatment goals. This chapter delves into critical aspects such as informed consent, ethical dilemmas in prescribing, the responsibilities of healthcare providers, and guidelines for deprescribing and managing end-of-life medications. By integrating patient-centered care, adherence to legal frameworks, and ethical decision-making, healthcare providers can address the multifaceted needs of elderly patients.

INFORMED CONSENT IN ELDERLY POPULATIONS

Informed consent is foundational to ethical and legal healthcare practices, ensuring that patients are aware of the implications, benefits, and risks of their treatment plans. For elderly patients, unique challenges such as cognitive decline, communication barriers, and complex medical conditions can complicate the consent process. A robust and patient-centered approach is necessary to navigate these challenges effectively.

COGNITIVE IMPAIRMENT

Elderly patients may suffer from conditions such as dementia, mild cognitive impairment (MCI), or other neurodegenerative diseases that limit their ability to understand complex medical information. This raises ethical concerns about their capacity to provide truly informed consent.

- *Role of legally authorized representatives:* When cognitive impairments preclude an elderly person from comprehending treatment details, consent must be obtained from legally authorized representatives, such as family members or court-appointed guardians. These representatives should be involved in care discussions and decision-making to ensure the patient's best interests are prioritized.

Example: Consider an elderly patient with moderate Alzheimer's disease being proposed for a surgical intervention. The healthcare team discusses the procedure, risks, and benefits with the patient's daughter, who is the designated legal guardian. The daughter's consent is documented, along with notes on the patient's limited cognitive capacity.

COMMUNICATION BARRIERS

Hearing loss, vision impairment, language difficulties, or even cultural factors can hinder effective communication with elderly patients. Tailored approaches to address these barriers are vital to ensure informed consent is genuinely informed.

- *Adaptations for sensory impairments*:
  - Use of large-font written materials for visually impaired patients.
  - Employing audio devices or written notes for those with hearing loss.
- *Language and cultural sensitivity:* For patients with language barriers, professional interpreters or culturally appropriate materials are necessary. Avoid relying on family members to interpret, as this can lead to misunderstandings or incomplete communication.

Example: A Bengali-speaking elderly patient requires consent for chemotherapy in Mumbai. The medical team arranges for a certified interpreter and uses pictorial aids to explain the treatment options. This ensures the patient comprehends the information and can make an informed choice.

CAPACITY ASSESSMENT

The capacity to consent is not static and may vary depending on the complexity of the decision and the patient's health status. Regular assessments of decision-making capacity are essential to validate the patient's ability to comprehend, reason, and communicate their choices.

- *Tools for assessment:* Instruments such as the Mini-Mental State Examination (MMSE) or the Montreal Cognitive Assessment (MoCA) can provide an objective measure of cognitive function.

- *Ethical considerations:* Healthcare providers must balance respecting autonomy with safeguarding the patient's welfare. Patients who lack full capacity for certain decisions might still contribute to discussions about less complex aspects of their care.

Example: An elderly patient with fluctuating cognitive function due to vascular dementia is presented with options for diabetes management. During a lucid period, the patient expresses a preference for lifestyle modifications over medication, which is respected and documented.

SHARED DECISION-MAKING

Shared decision-making (SDM) is an ethical approach that actively involves patients in their care planning, respecting their autonomy and preferences. For elderly patients, this approach is particularly important to align treatments with their goals, values, and quality of life.

- *Empowering elderly patients:* Even those with mild cognitive impairments can meaningfully participate in decisions if provided with clear and simple explanations.
- *Family involvement:* Including family members in discussions fosters trust and helps bridge gaps in understanding, provided that patient privacy and autonomy are respected.

Example: An elderly patient with chronic obstructive pulmonary disease (COPD) is offered the choice between continuing invasive therapies or transitioning to palliative care. The healthcare provider facilitates a meeting with the patient and their family to discuss the options, allowing the patient to voice preferences that are documented and respected.

CASE STUDY: INTEGRATING ETHICAL AND PRACTICAL SOLUTIONS

An 82-year-old patient with mild dementia is diagnosed with a serious but treatable infection requiring surgery. During discussions, the patient expresses concern about the risks and impact of surgery on their quality of life but struggles to understand the full implications. The healthcare provider:

- Uses simple language and diagrams to explain the procedure.
- Engages the patient's spouse, who holds durable power of attorney, to participate in the conversation.
- Conducts a cognitive assessment to confirm limited understanding.
- Documents the decision to proceed, supported by the spouse's consent, and includes the patient's expressed concerns.
- Ensuring informed consent for elderly patients is a nuanced process that requires sensitivity to cognitive, sensory, and communication challenges. By employing tailored approaches, involving family members appropriately, and maintaining a patient-centered focus, healthcare providers can uphold the principles of autonomy, beneficence, and justice in the care of elderly populations.

ETHICAL DILEMMAS IN PRESCRIBING FOR THE ELDERLY

Prescribing for elderly populations involves navigating a complex landscape of ethical dilemmas, arising from the interplay of chronic conditions, comorbidities, age-related physiological changes, and the varied goals of care. These dilemmas often center around balancing the risks and benefits of treatments while honoring the values and preferences of patients.

Overtreatment

Polypharmacy, or the use of multiple medications, is a common challenge in elderly care. While necessary in managing multiple conditions, it introduces significant risks:

- *Risks of polypharmacy:* Increased likelihood of adverse drug events (ADEs), such as falls, confusion, or gastrointestinal issues. Greater potential for drug-drug interactions, especially when medications are prescribed by different providers without comprehensive review. Increased pill burden, leading to non-adherence and reduced quality of life.
- *Strategies for ethical management:* Conduct regular medication reviews to assess the continued necessity of each drug. Prioritize deprescribing where possible, focusing on discontinuing medications that provide marginal benefits.

Example: An elderly patient with hypertension, diabetes, and arthritis is on ten medications. After a thorough review, the prescriber identifies that two medications for acid reflux and one for blood pressure are no longer essential. Reducing the regimen improves the patient's adherence and reduces side effects.

Undertreatment

In contrast, fear of adverse events may lead to undertreatment, where conditions such as pain, depression, or heart disease are inadequately managed. This can result in significant physical and psychological harm.

- *Impact of undertreatment:* Uncontrolled pain may lead to immobility, social isolation, and diminished quality of life. Untreated depression can exacerbate other chronic conditions and lead to increased healthcare utilization. Failing to address cardiovascular risks due to age bias may result in preventable morbidity.
- *Ethical responsibility:* Avoid ageism in prescribing decisions and treat patients based on their overall health status, not chronological age. Consider patient-reported outcomes to guide therapy decisions.

Example: A physician hesitates to prescribe an opioid for a 78-year-old patient with severe arthritis pain due to concerns about addiction. After discussing the patient's functional limitations and goals, a low-dose regimen is initiated with close monitoring, significantly improving the patient's mobility and mood.

BALANCING RISKS AND BENEFITS

The principle of proportionality underpins ethical prescribing—ensuring that the potential benefits of a treatment justify its risks. This balance is particularly critical in frail or terminally ill patients.

KEY CONSIDERATIONS

- Evaluate the life expectancy and how it aligns with the expected time to benefit from treatment.
- Account for the patient's frailty, as even minor side effects can have disproportionate impacts.
- Focus on interventions that enhance quality of life, rather than those aimed at long-term prevention.

Example: For a 90-year-old with advanced cancer, a statin for cardiovascular risk prevention is discontinued. Instead, the focus shifts to pain management and addressing nausea caused by chemotherapy, prioritizing comfort over preventative care.

PATIENT AUTONOMY VERSUS BENEFICENCE

Tensions frequently arise when patients' preferences conflict with what healthcare providers believe is in their best interests.

Autonomy

- Respecting the patient's right to refuse treatment, even if it may lead to adverse outcomes.
- Supporting informed decision-making by providing clear, unbiased information about risks and benefits.

Beneficence

- Acting in the patient's best interests when they lack the capacity to make informed decisions.
- Balancing the ethical obligation to protect patients from harm with the respect for their autonomy.

EXAMPLE OF CONFLICT

An elderly patient with severe heart failure refuses a recommended diuretic, citing unpleasant side effects. After discussing alternative options and explaining the potential consequences of not taking the medication, the patient decides to proceed with a reduced dose.

CASE STUDY: NAVIGATING ETHICAL DILEMMAS

An 85-year-old woman with chronic kidney disease and osteoporosis is prescribed several medications. Her family expresses concerns about the pill burden and side effects. The physician reviews her regimen and:

- Discontinues a bisphosphonate due to minimal expected benefit given her life expectancy.
- Initiates a shared decision-making (SDM) process to address her pain management preferences, balancing her reluctance to use strong painkillers with the need for mobility.

Ethical dilemmas in prescribing for the elderly highlight the need for personalized, patient-centered approaches. By addressing overtreatment and undertreatment, balancing risks and benefits, and navigating the tensions between autonomy and beneficence, healthcare providers can ensure care is both ethical and effective. Tailored strategies, open communication, and ongoing reviews are critical to achieving optimal outcomes for elderly patients.

LEGAL RESPONSIBILITIES OF PRESCRIBERS

Healthcare providers are bound by legal and professional standards to ensure the safety, dignity, and rights of elderly patients. These responsibilities encompass meticulous documentation, adherence to clinical guidelines, monitoring for adverse effects, and compliance with guardianship laws.

Documentation

Accurate and comprehensive documentation is a cornerstone of legal accountability in prescribing practices for elderly patients.

- *What to document*:
  - Rationale for prescribing decisions, including risk-benefit analyses.
  - Informed consent discussions, highlighting that the patient (or legal guardian) understood and agreed to the treatment plan.
  - Changes to treatment regimens, including reasons for initiating, discontinuing, or modifying medications.
  - Monitoring outcomes and adverse effects.
- *Legal importance*:
  - Thorough documentation protects prescribers in case of litigation or inquiries.
  - It provides a clear record for other healthcare providers involved in the patient's care.

Example: An elderly patient on anticoagulants experiences a gastrointestinal bleed. The physician's detailed documentation of prior discussions about the risks and benefits of anticoagulation therapy protects them during a subsequent legal review.

ADHERENCE TO GUIDELINES

Prescribers must align treatments with established local, national, or international guidelines to ensure that the care provided meets the standard of practice.

- *Importance of guideline adherence*:
  - Ensures evidence-based care, reducing variability and error.
  - Serves as a benchmark for legal and ethical scrutiny.
- *Challenges*:
  - Adapting guidelines for elderly patients with comorbidities or limited life expectancy.
  - Addressing areas where guidelines may be ambiguous or lacking.

Example: In managing hypertension, a prescriber follows updated guidelines to avoid aggressive treatment targets in frail elderly patients, focusing instead on preventing falls and adverse events.

MONITORING AND REPORTING

Monitoring elderly patients for adverse drug reactions (ADRs) and reporting medication errors are legal and ethical obligations for healthcare providers.

- *Monitoring*:
  - Regular assessments of drug efficacy and tolerability.
  - Adjusting dosages based on physiological changes such as renal or hepatic impairment.
- *Reporting requirements*: Prescribers must report serious ADRs to regulatory bodies such as the PVPI (Pharmacovigilance Programme of India).

Example: After initiating a new antipsychotic medication in a patient with dementia, a prescriber detects severe sedation and reports the adverse reaction to improve drug safety monitoring.

GUARDIANSHIP LAWS

When elderly patients cannot provide informed consent, legal frameworks for substituted decision-making guide care decisions.

- *Substituted decision-making options*:
  - *Advance directives:* Documents specifying the patient's preferences for future medical care.
  - *Living wills:* Instructions for care in terminal or irreversible conditions.
  - *Durable power of attorney:* Designates a proxy to make healthcare decisions.
- *Prescriber responsibility*:
  - Verify the legal validity of decision-making documents.
  - Collaborate with proxies to align care with the patient's values and preferences.

Example: A patient in a persistent vegetative state has an advance directive refusing artificial nutrition. The prescriber consults with the family and legal advisors to honor the directive.

GUIDELINES FOR MANAGING END-OF-LIFE MEDICATIONS

Managing medications for patients at the end of life requires balancing symptom control, ethical principles, and legal obligations. The primary goal is to prioritize the patient's comfort and quality of life.

- *Palliative intent*: Medications in end-of-life care should aim to relieve symptoms rather than cure underlying conditions.
- *Focus areas*:
  - Pain management (e.g., opioids for severe pain)
  - Symptom relief, such as anti-nausea drugs or bronchodilators for breathlessness.

- *Avoiding overtreatment*: Discontinue therapies with no short-term benefits, such as statins or osteoporosis treatments.

Example: For a patient with terminal cancer, the physician shifts focus from chemotherapy to high-dose opioids for pain relief and low-dose benzodiazepines for anxiety.

Proportionality

Symptom relief should be balanced against the risks of over-sedation or diminished quality of life.

- *Ethical sedation*:
  - Use the minimum effective dose to manage symptoms such as severe agitation or respiratory distress.
  - Avoid excessive sedation unless clinically justified for refractory symptoms.

Example: In a dying patient with severe dyspnea, the prescriber uses titrated morphine doses to relieve discomfort without causing undue sedation.

Advance Care Planning

Discussions about care goals are essential for aligning end-of-life treatment with the patient's wishes.

- *Components*:
  - Clarifying whether the patient wants aggressive interventions, such as resuscitation or intubation.
  - Exploring preferences for pain management and symptom relief.
- *Family involvement*: Engaging families ensure that care decisions respect both the patient's and the family's perspectives.

Example: A patient with advanced dementia has a family discussion facilitated by the physician, resulting in a consensus to focus on hospice care.

Withdrawal of Medications

Discontinuing non-essential or harmful medications is an ethical aspect of end-of-life care.

- *Considerations*:
  - Stop treatments unlikely to provide immediate benefits (e.g., cholesterol-lowering drugs).
  - Focus on simplifying medication regimens to reduce burden and enhance comfort.

Example: In a terminally ill patient with diabetes, the prescriber discontinues long-acting insulin while continuing short-acting insulin to manage symptomatic hyperglycemia.

Legal responsibilities and guidelines for managing end-of-life medications require prescribers to maintain a meticulous balance between ethical, medical, and legal considerations. By adhering to robust documentation practices, monitoring and reporting protocols, and focusing on patient-centered care, prescribers can uphold their duties while delivering compassionate and effective treatment.

GUIDELINES FOR MANAGING END-OF-LIFE MEDICATIONS

End-of-life care focuses on ensuring comfort and dignity for patients as they face terminal conditions. Prescribing at this stage requires careful balancing of symptom management, ethical considerations, and legal obligations. These guidelines aim to prioritize the patient's quality of life while addressing the complexities of treatment withdrawal and palliative care.

Palliative Intent

Medications at the end of life should aim to alleviate symptoms rather than cure the underlying disease.

- *Focus areas*:
    - *Pain management:* Opioids such as morphine or hydromorphone are frequently used to manage severe pain effectively.
    - *Symptom relief:* Medications such as antiemetics (e.g., ondansetron) for nausea or bronchodilators for breathlessness may be prioritized.
    - *Anxiety and restlessness:* Sedatives such as benzodiazepines are often employed to address psychological distress.
- *Avoiding aggressive therapies*: Treatments such as chemotherapy, dialysis, or intensive glucose control are often inappropriate at this stage and should be avoided unless they contribute directly to symptom relief.

Example: A patient with metastatic cancer is prescribed a combination of opioids for pain and low-dose lorazepam for anxiety. Chemotherapy is discontinued due to its minimal benefit and potential for causing distressing side effects.

Proportionality

The principle of proportionality ensures that medications used to relieve symptoms do not unduly compromise the patient's quality of life by causing excessive sedation or other adverse effects.

- *Titrated symptom management*:
    - Medications should be started at the lowest effective dose and titrated based on the patient's response.
    - Avoid "blanket" sedation unless symptoms are refractory to other interventions.
- *Ethical sedation*: In cases of intractable symptoms such as severe dyspnea or agitation, palliative sedation may be appropriate. However, the goal is to relieve suffering, not to hasten death.

Example: A terminally ill patient with uncontrolled dyspnea is administered low-dose morphine for relief. If the dyspnea persists, the dose is increased incrementally until the patient achieves comfort without significant respiratory depression.

ADVANCE CARE PLANNING

Advance care planning (ACP) is essential for aligning the goals of care with the patient's values, preferences, and medical needs.

- *Key components*:
  - *Goals of care:* Discuss whether the focus is on comfort, life extension, or a combination of both.
  - *Pain management:* Ensure patients and families understand available options for controlling pain and other distressing symptoms.
  - *Life-sustaining treatments:* Clarify preferences regarding interventions such as resuscitation, mechanical ventilation, or tube feeding.
- *Family involvement*: Families often play a crucial role in decision-making, especially when patients cannot articulate their preferences. Open communication reduces misunderstandings and aligns care with the patient's values.

Example: An elderly patient with advanced COPD discusses their preference to avoid intubation during respiratory crises. This preference is documented in an advance directive and communicated to the care team.

WITHDRAWAL OF MEDICATIONS

As patients near the end of life, many medications aimed at long-term benefits are no longer appropriate and should be ethically discontinued.

- *Key considerations*:
  - *Evaluate necessity:* Medications such as statins, antihypertensives, and osteoporosis treatments may provide minimal benefit in the remaining lifespan.
  - *Minimize burden:* Simplifying the medication regimen can improve the patient's comfort and reduce unnecessary side effects.
  - *Patient-centered decisions:* Discussing medication withdrawal with patients and families ensures transparency and respects the patient's autonomy.
- *Ethical justification*: Discontinuing non-essential medications aligns with the principles of beneficence (acting in the patient's best interest) and non-maleficence (avoiding harm).

Example: A patient with advanced dementia and limited life expectancy is tapered off statins and antihypertensives. The focus shifts to comfort measures, including low-dose opioids and antipsychotics for agitation.

PRACTICAL CONSIDERATIONS AND IMPLEMENTATION

- *Regular reassessment*: As the patient's condition evolves, reassess the effectiveness and appropriateness of all prescribed medications.
- *Interdisciplinary approach*: Involve palliative care specialists, pharmacists, and nurses to develop a comprehensive care plan.
- *Cultural sensitivity*: Tailor discussions and care plans to the cultural beliefs and values of the patient and their family.

End-of-life prescribing demands a delicate balance between providing effective symptom relief and avoiding unnecessary interventions. By focusing on palliative intent, maintaining proportionality in symptom management, engaging in ACP, and ethically withdrawing non-essential medications, healthcare providers can uphold the dignity and comfort of patients during this critical phase of care.

ETHICAL CONSIDERATIONS IN DEPRESCRIBING

Deprescribing is an essential process in the management of elderly patients, aimed at optimizing medication use by discontinuing those that are unnecessary, ineffective, or potentially harmful. This practice not only minimizes ADEs but also aligns treatment regimens with the patient's evolving health goals and quality of life.

Holistic Review

A comprehensive review of the patient's medication regimen is the first step in deprescribing.

- *Components of review*:
  - Identify medications with marginal benefits or those prescribed for conditions no longer relevant to the patient's health.
  - Assess drugs with high potential for adverse effects or drug-drug interactions, especially in polypharmacy settings.
  - Consider the patient's current goals of care, such as transitioning from curative to palliative treatments.

Example: An 80-year-old patient taking a bisphosphonate for osteoporosis is bedbound and unlikely to benefit from fracture prevention. The drug is identified as a candidate for deprescribing after assessing risks and benefits.

Patient-centered Approach

Engaging patients and caregivers in discussions about deprescribing is crucial to ensure understanding, build trust, and address concerns.

- *Communication strategies*:
  - Clearly explain the rationale for deprescribing, emphasizing how it reduces risks and aligns with the patient's care goals.
  - Address fears of symptom recurrence or withdrawal effects to alleviate patient anxiety.
  - Involve caregivers to ensure SDM and support adherence.

Example: A patient expresses concern about stopping a proton pump inhibitor (PPI) used for gastroesophageal reflux disease despite no recent symptoms. The prescriber explains that continuing the PPI unnecessarily increases the risk of osteoporosis and ensures the patient that symptoms will be monitored closely after cessation.

Gradual Process

Abrupt discontinuation of medications can lead to withdrawal syndromes or exacerbation of underlying conditions. A gradual tapering strategy is often the safest approach.

- *Principles of tapering*:
  - For medications such as benzodiazepines or antidepressants, a slow reduction in dose over weeks or months can prevent withdrawal symptoms.
  - Use a stepwise approach, prioritizing the cessation of high-risk drugs first.

Example: A long-term benzodiazepine user with insomnia undergoes a tapering schedule, starting with a 25% dose reduction every 2 weeks. The patient is also provided with non-pharmacologic interventions for sleep management, such as cognitive behavioral therapy.

Monitoring

Post-deprescribing monitoring is critical to evaluate the impact of discontinuation on the patient's health and to address any emerging issues.

- *What to monitor*:
  - Changes in symptoms or the recurrence of the condition the medication was managing.
  - Signs of withdrawal, particularly for medications affecting the central nervous system (e.g., opioids, antidepressants).
  - General well-being and quality of life indicators.
- *Adjustment of care plans*: Reintroduce medications if clinically necessary, or explore alternative therapies if symptoms persist or worsen.

Example: After stopping a diuretic in a patient with mild heart failure, the prescriber monitors for signs of fluid retention and educates the patient about early symptoms to report, such as swelling or shortness of breath.

ETHICAL IMPLICATIONS

Deprescribing raises ethical considerations that require careful balancing of risks and benefits, with an emphasis on the patient's autonomy and clinical context.

- *Balancing risks*:
  - Continuing unnecessary medications can expose patients to harm, including falls, cognitive impairment, and organ toxicity.
  - Cessation, however, may pose risks such as symptom recurrence or loss of perceived stability.
- *Respecting autonomy*: Deprescribing decisions should prioritize the patient's preferences, values, and quality of life, particularly in palliative or end-of-life care settings.

Example: In a terminally ill patient with no clinical benefit from statins, the prescriber discusses stopping the medication to reduce pill burden, improving the patient's overall experience without compromising their comfort.

PRACTICAL CONSIDERATIONS IN DEPRESCRIBING

- *Interdisciplinary approach:* Involve pharmacists, nurses, and other healthcare providers to ensure a coordinated and thorough review of the medication regimen.

- *Education and awareness:* Educate patients and families about the importance of deprescribing in minimizing risks and improving quality of life.
- *Tailored strategies:* Recognize that deprescribing is not a one-size-fits-all process. Individualized care plans should be based on the patient's specific needs and health status.

Deprescribing is not just a clinical task but an ethical obligation to ensure that elderly patients receive appropriate, safe, and effective care. By conducting holistic reviews, engaging patients and caregivers, using gradual processes, and monitoring outcomes, healthcare providers can navigate the complexities of deprescribing while upholding ethical standards. This approach not only enhances patient safety but also improves their overall quality of life.

The recommendations as depicted in **Box 1**, for ethical and legal considerations in prescribing for the elderly emphasize a patient-centered, evidence-based approach to medication management. Comprehensive medication reviews are crucial for identifying drugs that may no longer be necessary, ineffective, or potentially harmful, with a focus on deprescribing where appropriate. Ensuring informed consent tailored to the cognitive and sensory challenges of elderly patients is essential, incorporating tools such as visual aids, interpreters, and clear communication. SDM empowers patients and their families, aligning medical interventions with individual values and care goals. Addressing polypharmacy risks by streamlining treatments and prioritizing medications with clear benefits can mitigate adverse effects and improve adherence. Avoiding undertreatment is equally important, ensuring conditions such as pain, depression, and cardiovascular diseases are adequately managed based on functional health rather than age. Accurate documentation of prescribing decisions protects both patients and prescribers and supports accountability. Adherence to clinical guidelines tailored to the elderly population, especially those with comorbidities or limited life expectancy, ensures evidence-based care. For end-of-life prescribing, the focus should shift to palliative intent, emphasizing comfort and proportional symptom relief over aggressive treatments. A gradual, monitored deprescribing process avoids withdrawal effects and maintains patient stability, while respecting legal and ethical obligations, including guardianship laws and advance directives, ensures that care aligns with the patient's best interests and documented wishes. These strategies collectively promote safe, ethical, and effective prescribing for the elderly.

CONCLUSION

Prescribing for the elderly is a delicate balance of clinical, ethical, and legal considerations. It demands a comprehensive, patient-centered approach that addresses informed consent, ethical dilemmas in over- and undertreatment, deprescribing practices, and end-of-life care. By upholding the principles of autonomy, beneficence, and justice, while adhering to legal frameworks, healthcare providers can deliver compassionate, effective, and ethically sound care. Tailored interventions, ongoing communication with patients and families, and an interdisciplinary approach are key to optimizing outcomes and enhancing the quality of life for elderly patients.

BOX 1 Recommendations for ethical and legal considerations in prescribing for the elderly.

- *Comprehensive medication review*: Regularly assess all medications in an elderly patient's regimen to identify those that are unnecessary, ineffective, or potentially harmful. Focus on deprescribing medications with marginal benefits or high risk of adverse effects
- *Ensure informed consent*: Tailor the consent process to accommodate cognitive and sensory challenges in elderly patients. Use simple language, visual aids, interpreters, or large-font documents to ensure comprehension and active participation in decision-making
- *Empower shared decision-making*: Actively involve elderly patients and their families in treatment planning. Respect autonomy by aligning medical interventions with the patient's values, preferences, and goals of care
- *Address polypharmacy risks*: Mitigate risks of polypharmacy by implementing evidence-based strategies to streamline treatment. Prioritize medications that provide clear benefits while reducing the overall pill burden
- *Avoid undertreatment*: Counteract age-related bias by ensuring adequate management of conditions such as pain, depression, and cardiovascular diseases. Base treatment decisions on functional health status rather than chronological age
- *Document prescribing decisions*: Maintain detailed and accurate records of prescribing decisions, informed consent discussions, and rationales for changes in medication regimens. This protects both patients and prescribers in case of legal disputes
- *Adhere to clinical guidelines*: Stay informed about current best practices and adapt clinical guidelines to address the specific needs of elderly patients with comorbidities and limited life expectancy. Strive for evidence-based care tailored to individual circumstances
- *Prioritize palliative intent in end-of-life care*: Focus end-of-life prescribing on comfort and quality of life. Avoid unnecessary or aggressive treatments that do not align with the patient's goals and use proportional interventions to manage symptoms effectively
- *Gradual and monitored deprescribing*: Implement a systematic, gradual tapering approach for discontinuing medications to avoid withdrawal effects and rebound symptoms. Monitor patient outcomes closely and adjust treatment plans as needed
- *Respect legal and ethical obligations*: Familiarize yourself with guardianship laws, advance directives, and other legal frameworks governing decision-making for elderly patients. Collaborate with legally authorized representatives to align care with the patient's best interests and documented wishes

SUGGESTED READINGS

1. Khalil H. Prescribing for the elderly: ethical considerations. Aust J Prim Health. 2011;17(1):2-3.
2. Santos Cruz R, Brito-Costa S, Santa Rosa B, Silvestre M. Overtreatment in elderly care: ethical considerations. Acta Biomed. 2022;93(2):e2022136.
3. Norton JD, Zeng C, Bayliss EA, Shetterly SM, Williams N, Reeve E, et al. Ethical Aspects of Physician Decision-Making for Deprescribing Among Older Adults with Dementia. JAMA Netw Open. 2023;6(10):e2336728.
4. Alodhialah AM, Almutairi AA, Almutairi M. Ethical and legal challenges in caring for older adults with multimorbidities: Best practices for nurses. Healthcare. 2024;12(16):1585.

8

CHAPTER

Rational Prescribing and Medication Management in Elderly Patients: Case Studies in Evidence-based Practices and Adverse Reaction Mitigation

ABSTRACT

Rational prescribing in elderly patients is crucial for balancing effective treatment with the prevention of adverse drug reactions (ADRs) and healthcare overuse. This chapter presents three case studies that highlight evidence-based approaches to managing asymptomatic bacteriuria (ASB), ensuring accurate drug dosing through estimated glomerular filtration rate (eGFR) calculations, and recognizing ADRs in the context of polypharmacy. These cases emphasize the importance of avoiding unnecessary antibiotic use in ASB to prevent antimicrobial resistance, tailoring drug regimens based on precise renal function assessments to minimize toxicity, and identifying drug-induced symptoms using tools like the Anticholinergic Cognitive Burden (ACB) scale to prevent prescribing cascades. By adhering to clinical guidelines, conducting systematic medication reviews, and fostering antimicrobial and pharmacological stewardship, healthcare providers can enhance patient safety, optimize therapeutic outcomes, and address broader challenges such as antibiotic resistance and polypharmacy-related complications. These examples underscore the need for patient-centered, evidence-based practices in elderly care to improve outcomes and promote safer prescribing.

INTRODUCTION

Rational prescribing in elderly patients is a cornerstone of geriatric medicine, balancing the need for effective treatment with the prevention of adverse drug reactions (ADRs) and healthcare overuse. With age, physiological changes such as reduced renal function, altered drug metabolism, and increased susceptibility to polypharmacy complicate the safe and effective use of medications. These complexities necessitate evidence-based approaches to prescribing that consider individual patient characteristics, clinical scenarios, and the risks associated with overtreatment or mismanagement.

Elderly patients are uniquely vulnerable to the consequences of inappropriate medication use. Overprescription, often due to misinterpretation of clinical findings or a failure to recognize age-related physiological changes, can lead to significant harms such as antimicrobial resistance, drug toxicities, and cascading medical complications. Conversely, under-recognition of ADRs or disease progression can result in missed treatment opportunities, exacerbating patient morbidity and healthcare costs.

This collection of case studies highlights three critical aspects of rational prescribing in the elderly:

- *Managing asymptomatic bacteriuria (ASB):* Emphasizing the importance of avoiding unnecessary antibiotic use in asymptomatic elderly individuals to prevent antimicrobial resistance and adverse effects.
- *Accurate estimated glomerular filtration rate (eGFR) calculation before prescribing:* Demonstrating the significance of renal function assessment in tailoring drug dosing and preventing toxicity.
- *Recognizing ADRs:* Addressing the challenge of distinguishing drug-induced symptoms from disease progression in the context of polypharmacy.

Each case underscores the importance of a patient-centered, evidence-based approach to medication management. By adhering to clinical guidelines, conducting thorough assessments, and fostering a culture of stewardship, healthcare providers can enhance patient safety, optimize therapeutic outcomes, and mitigate the broader public health challenges associated with medication misuse in the elderly. These case studies serve as practical examples of how thoughtful prescribing can improve care for this vulnerable population.

CASE STUDY 1: RATIONAL PRESCRIBING IN ELDERLY PATIENTS: MANAGING ASYMPTOMATIC BACTERIURIA

Knowing When Not to Prescribe: A Rational Approach to Asymptomatic Bacteriuria in the Elderly

Introduction

Antibiotics are often overprescribed for ASB, particularly in elderly populations, where routine urine cultures frequently reveal the presence of bacteria without clinical symptoms. This overprescription contributes significantly to antibiotic resistance, ADRs, and avoidable healthcare expenses. This case study delves into evidence-based guidelines to avoid unnecessary treatment of ASB in older adults, exploring the risks of inappropriate prescribing and highlighting the benefits of rational decision-making.

Patient Background

- *Name:* Mrs TKS
- *Age:* 85 years
- *Residence:* Long-term care facility
- *Medical history:* Cognitive impairment, type 2 diabetes mellitus (T2DM), osteoarthritis, and a history of recurrent urinary tract infections (UTIs).
- *Current symptoms*: None

Routine screening during an annual health evaluation detected bacteriuria with *Escherichia coli* (*E. coli*) >10^5 CFU/mL. Despite the findings, Mrs TKS exhibited no genitourinary symptoms (e.g., dysuria, urgency, or flank pain), systemic signs of infection (e.g., fever, hemodynamic instability), or cognitive changes beyond her baseline impairment.

Clinical Scenario

The detection of bacteriuria in asymptomatic individuals often leads to unnecessary antibiotic therapy. In this case, however, the care team adhered to evidence-based guidelines, opting for close monitoring instead of initiating treatment. This decision aimed to avoid exposing the patient to potential harms associated with unwarranted antibiotic use while safeguarding her health through appropriate observation.

Clinical Guidelines and Evidence-based Approach

Key Recommendations

- *Do not treat asymptomatic bacteriuria without symptoms:* Evidence consistently demonstrates that treating ASB in elderly patients without symptoms provides no clinical benefit. It does not reduce the risk of UTIs, improve quality of life, or lower mortality rates.
- *Avoid routine screening for asymptomatic bacteriuria:* Routine urine cultures in the absence of symptoms are not recommended for elderly patients in long-term care settings due to their low clinical utility and high risk of overtreatment.
- *Monitor for symptomatic urinary tract infection:* Treatment should only be initiated if clear signs of infection, such as fever, dysuria, flank pain, or hemodynamic instability, develop.

Potential Harm from Antibiotic Misuse in Asymptomatic Bacteriuria

Promotes Antibiotic Resistance

- *Mechanism:* Antibiotics exert selective pressure on bacteria, fostering the survival and multiplication of resistant strains. This is particularly concerning for gram-negative pathogens such as *E. coli* and *Klebsiella pneumoniae*, which are common in ASB.
- *Clinical consequences:* Multidrug-resistant organisms (MDROs) such as ESBL-producing *E. coli* or carbapenem-resistant *Enterobacterales* (CRE) complicate future treatment options, increasing morbidity and healthcare costs.

Increases Risk of Recurrent Symptomatic Urinary Tract Infections

- *Impact:* Treating ASB disrupts the urinary microbiome, making patients more susceptible to recurrent infections caused by resistant pathogens.
- *Outcome*: Recurrent UTIs in elderly patients are more likely to require hospitalization, invasive procedures, and costly second-line antibiotics.

Adverse Drug Reactions

- *Gastrointestinal effects:* Antibiotics can cause diarrhea, dehydration, and malnutrition in frail elderly patients.
- *Clostridioides difficile (C. difficile) infection (CDI):* Broad-spectrum antibiotics disrupt gut flora, leading to overgrowth of *C. difficile*. CDI is associated with high morbidity and mortality, especially in older adults.

- *Hypersensitivity reactions:* Elderly patients are at increased risk of severe hypersensitivity, such as Stevens–Johnson syndrome or toxic epidermal necrolysis.
- *Organ toxicity:* Renal and hepatic adverse effects can be life-threatening in patients with diminished organ reserve.

Management and Outcomes

Action Taken

- *Refraining from antibiotics:* The care team, adhering to evidence-based guidelines, decided against prescribing antibiotics. Instead, they monitored Mrs TKS for potential signs of symptomatic infection.
- *Education for healthcare staff:* Staff members were educated on distinguishing ASB from symptomatic UTIs, emphasizing the importance of avoiding unnecessary urine culture requests in asymptomatic patients.

Outcome

- *Patient-specific results*: Over a 6-month observation period, Mrs TKS remained asymptomatic with no signs of infection or complications. Her health and quality of life were unaffected, affirming the safety of withholding treatment for ASB.
- *Institutional impact*:
  - *Reduction in antibiotic use:* The facility achieved a 30% reduction in antibiotic prescriptions for ASB, minimizing the risk of CDI and antimicrobial resistance.
  - *Enhanced stewardship:* By avoiding unnecessary testing and treatment, the institution fostered a culture of evidence-based decision-making, improving patient care and reducing healthcare costs.

Discussion

This case underscores the critical importance of adhering to evidence-based clinical guidelines in managing ASB among elderly patients. Treating ASB unnecessarily exposes patients to significant risks, including ADRs, antibiotic resistance, and recurrent infections. In contrast, withholding treatment in asymptomatic cases aligns with best practices, ensuring better patient outcomes and promoting antimicrobial stewardship.

Avoidance of Potential Harm

- *Adverse drug reactions:* The decision to refrain from antibiotics protected Mrs TKS from gastrointestinal side effects, CDI, and hypersensitivity reactions.
- *Resistance development:* Antibiotic misuse is a leading cause of MDRO proliferation, complicating future infection management.
- *Healthcare burden:* By avoiding unwarranted treatment, the facility-reduced hospital stays, diagnostic costs, and overall healthcare expenditures.

Promotion of Antimicrobial Stewardship

The case demonstrates how rational prescribing at the individual level drives systemic improvements. By educating staff and standardizing care protocols, the facility achieved significant institutional benefits, including enhanced patient safety, better resource utilization, and reduced rates of antibiotic resistance.

Broader Implications for Practice

- *Educating healthcare providers:* Training on the distinction between ASB and symptomatic UTIs is essential to avoid unnecessary interventions.
- *Standardizing protocols:* Implementing evidence-based guidelines for ASB management can reduce inappropriate antibiotic use and associated harms.
- *Fostering stewardship:* Rational prescribing supports broader public health goals, preserving the efficacy of antibiotics and reducing resistance rates.

Conclusion

This case study illustrates the importance of rational prescribing in managing ASB in elderly populations. By adhering to evidence-based guidelines, the care team successfully avoided unnecessary antibiotic use for Mrs TKS, safeguarding her from potential harms such as ADRs, CDI, and antimicrobial resistance. The decision not to treat ASB not only benefited Mrs TKS but also catalyzed broader institutional improvements in antimicrobial stewardship. This approach highlights the need for evidence-based practices that prioritize patient safety, uphold antibiotic efficacy, and minimize public health risks.

By embracing these principles, healthcare providers can ensure better outcomes for patients while addressing the growing challenge of antibiotic resistance.

CASE STUDY 2: RATIONAL PRESCRIBING IN ELDERLY PATIENTS: IMPORTANCE OF CALCULATING ESTIMATED GLOMERULAR FILTRATION RATE BEFORE PRESCRIBING

Precision in Prescribing: The Role of Estimated Glomerular Filtration Rate in Preventing Adverse Outcomes in Elderly Patients

Introduction

Prescribing medications in elderly patients requires a careful balance between therapeutic benefit and the potential for harm. Many drugs are eliminated through the kidneys, and age-related physiological changes, particularly in renal function, demand precision in drug dosing. Estimated glomerular filtration rate (eGFR) is a cornerstone of assessing kidney function, but improper calculation can lead to ADRs, therapeutic failure, and unnecessary healthcare burdens. This case study explores the importance of accurate eGFR assessment, highlighting its role in preventing complications and ensuring safe prescribing for elderly patients.

Patient Background

- *Name:* Mrs RG
- *Age:* 75 years

- *Residence:* Assisted living facility
- *Medical history:* Chronic kidney disease (CKD), type 2 diabetes mellitus (T2DM), hypertension (HTN), and a recent ischemic stroke.
- *Clinical presentation:* Hospitalized for stroke management, serum creatinine level measured at 1.9 mg/dL.

Clinical Scenario

Mrs RG was admitted to the critical care unit following a lacunar infarct affecting her left hemisphere. During her stay, an empiric antibiotic regimen of imipenem-cilastatin was initiated to manage a suspected hospital-acquired infection. Drug dosing was calculated using the chronic kidney disease-epidemiology collaboration (CKD-EPI) equation, yielding an eGFR of 35.1 mL/min/1.73 m^2. Based on this estimate, she was prescribed imipenem-cilastatin at a standard dosing interval of 500 mg every 8 hours.

However, within 48 hours of initiating the treatment, Mrs RG experienced generalized tonic-clonic seizures (GTCS). This adverse event raised concerns about potential drug toxicity. Upon recalculating renal function using the Cockcroft–Gault formula, her eGFR was found to be significantly lower, at 25.85 mL/min/1.73 m^2. The discrepancy in eGFR highlighted an error in dosing frequency, necessitating immediate correction. Imipenem-cilastatin was discontinued, and her seizures were managed with supportive care.

Clinical Guidelines and Evidence-based Approach

Key Recommendations for Renal Dosing in the Elderly

- *Select the appropriate eGFR formula:* The CKD-EPI equation is suitable for staging CKD but may overestimate renal function in elderly patients with reduced muscle mass. The Cockcroft–Gault formula, which incorporates weight and serum creatinine, is preferred for drug dosing, especially in frail individuals.
- *Adjust dosing for renally cleared medications:* Many drugs, including antibiotics such as imipenem-cilastatin, require dose adjustments to match the patient's actual renal clearance. Failure to dose appropriately can result in accumulation, increasing the risk of drug toxicity.
- *Incorporate clinical pharmacological reconciliation:* Regularly review the patient's medication regimen, considering renal function, polypharmacy, and comorbidities. Monitor renal function dynamically, as acute changes in creatinine clearance can alter dosing requirements.

Potential Harm from Incorrect Estimated Glomerular Filtration Rate Calculation

Risk of Adverse Drug Reactions

- *Neurotoxicity:* Imipenem, when overdosed in patients with renal impairment, can cross the blood-brain barrier and cause central nervous system toxicity, manifesting as seizures or encephalopathy.
- *Systemic toxicity:* Accumulation of renally eliminated drugs increases the risk of other organ dysfunction, including hepatotoxicity and cardiotoxicity.

Development of a Prescribing Cascade

Incorrect eGFR estimation and subsequent overdosing can trigger adverse events, leading to the addition of unnecessary medications.

In Mrs RG's case, her seizures might have led to prescribing benzodiazepines or anticonvulsants, potentially causing sedation, respiratory depression, or further complications.

Impact on Healthcare Resources

- *Extended hospital stays:* Adverse drug reactions require additional diagnostic and therapeutic interventions, delaying discharge and increasing costs.
- *Increased costs:* Managing complications from inappropriate drug dosing can lead to higher utilization of healthcare resources, including intensive care and monitoring.

Management and Outcomes

Action Taken

- *Recalculation of eGFR:* Using the Cockcroft-Gault formula, her eGFR was recalculated as 25.85 mL/min/1.73 m^2. This revealed significant renal impairment, necessitating a change in dosing. The imipenem-cilastatin dose was adjusted to 500 mg every 12 hours instead of every 8 hours to match her renal clearance capacity.
- *Discontinuation of imipenem-cilastatin:* Once it was identified as the likely cause of seizures, the antibiotic was stopped. An alternative regimen less dependent on renal clearance was initiated.
- *Supportive management:* Mrs RG's seizures were treated symptomatically with a short course of benzodiazepines. No chronic anticonvulsant therapy was required.
- *Education and protocol development:* The care team reviewed hospital policies to mandate eGFR calculations using the Cockcroft-Gault formula for elderly patients (as per prescribing information). A multidisciplinary team was established to review medication regimens for elderly patients with CKD.

Outcome

- *Patient recovery:* Mrs RG's seizures resolved, and she remained afebrile and clinically stable after discontinuing the offending medication. Her condition improved steadily, and she was discharged in stable health.
- *Institutional improvements:* The facility observed a significant reduction in adverse drug events following protocol changes, promoting safer prescribing practices for elderly patients.

Discussion

This case highlights the critical role of precision in drug dosing for elderly patients. Renal function estimation is not only essential for managing CKD but also for tailoring medication regimens. Misestimating eGFR can lead to overdosing, resulting in adverse outcomes such as drug-induced seizures and cascading medical complications.

The Cockcroft-Gault formula remains a reliable tool for renal dosing adjustments for drugs such as imipenem, as it accounts for body weight and is more accurate in frail, elderly individuals. This approach ensures that renally excreted drugs such as imipenem are dosed appropriately, reducing the risk of toxicity and improving clinical outcomes.

Beyond individual care, the case underscores the importance of institutional policies and education. By standardizing eGFR calculations and fostering a culture of pharmacological reconciliation, healthcare facilities can enhance patient safety, minimize adverse events, and optimize resource utilization.

Broader Implications for Practice

- *Promoting patient safety:* Tailored drug dosing based on accurate eGFR calculations prevents toxicity, particularly in vulnerable elderly populations.
- *Enhancing clinical outcomes:* Correct prescribing minimizes complications, reduces hospitalization duration, and improves recovery rates.
- *Strengthening antimicrobial stewardship:* Avoiding inappropriate antibiotic dosing supports broader public health goals of minimizing resistance and preserving the efficacy of critical drugs.
- *Implementing continuous education:* Ongoing training for healthcare providers on renal pharmacokinetics is essential to ensure compliance with best practices.

Conclusion

The case of Mrs RG underscores the importance of accurately calculating eGFR in elderly patients to ensure safe prescribing. Missteps in renal dosing can lead to serious complications, including neurotoxicity and cascading medical interventions. By integrating precise eGFR assessment, such as the Cockcroft-Gault formula, into routine care and fostering a culture of clinical pharmacological vigilance, healthcare providers can enhance patient safety and outcomes. This case serves as a vital reminder of the need for evidence-based, individualized approaches in managing the complexities of elderly patient care.

CASE STUDY 3: RECOGNIZING ADVERSE DRUG REACTIONS IN THE ELDERLY THROUGH PROGRESSION OF DISEASE

Distinguishing Adverse Drug Reactions from Disease Progression in Geriatric Care

Introduction

Adverse drug reactions are a common yet often underrecognized challenge in elderly care. As older adults frequently present with complex medical histories and polypharmacy, distinguishing between disease progression and drug-induced symptoms is crucial for effective management. Failure to identify ADRs can lead to misdiagnosis, unnecessary interventions, and increased morbidity. This case study explores the importance of recognizing ADRs in the context of polypharmacy, emphasizing the need for systematic medication review and vigilance in clinical assessment.

Patient Background

- *Name:* Mrs ZB
- *Age:* 66 years
- *Residence:* Community dwelling
- *Medical history:* Hypertension, major depression, alcohol abuse, and chronic tinea cruris
- *Current medications:*
  - Venlafaxine 150 mg daily for depression
  - Losartan 50 mg twice daily for hypertension
  - Terbinafine 500 mg daily for tinea cruris

Clinical Scenario

Mrs ZB presented to the emergency department (ED) with a sudden onset of altered mental status. Her family reported confusion, disorientation, and episodes of slurred speech over the past 24 hours. Additional complaints included visual hallucinations, dryness of the mouth, and difficulty urinating.

Physical Examination Findings

- *Blood pressure:* 180/102 mm Hg
- *Heart rate:* 120 beats/min (tachycardia)
- *Temperature:* Normal
- *Oxygen saturation:* 98% on room air
- *Pupils:* Dilated and sluggishly reactive
- *Skin:* Flushed and dry
- *Neurological examination:* No focal deficits but marked agitation and restlessness
- *Initial considerations:* The presentation raised concerns for a central nervous system (CNS) disorder, with differential diagnoses including stroke, delirium secondary to systemic infection, and potential drug toxicity.

Investigations and Findings

- *Initial laboratory tests*:
  - *Blood counts, electrolytes, and metabolic panel:* Unremarkable
  - *Urinalysis:* No evidence of infection
  - *Serum creatinine:* Normal, ruling out acute kidney injury
  - *Liver function tests:* Within normal limits
- *Medication review:* A thorough history revealed that Mrs ZB had been self-medicating with promethazine 25 mg, purchased over the counter, multiple times daily for pruritus associated with her tinea cruris. This medication, in combination with her prescribed drugs, contributed to a high anticholinergic burden.
- *Diagnosis:* Anticholinergic toxidrome clinical features, including tachycardia, urinary retention, dilated pupils, dry mucosa, and altered mental status,

pointed to anticholinergic toxicity as the primary cause of her presentation. The excessive use of promethazine, coupled with her regular medications, created a cumulative anticholinergic load.

Clinical Guidelines and Evidence-based Approach

Key Recommendations

- *Holistic medication review*:
  - Collect a complete medication history, including over-the-counter drugs and herbal remedies.
  - Evaluate cumulative anticholinergic effects using tools such as the Anticholinergic Cognitive Burden (ACB) scale.
- *Use of diagnostic frameworks*:
  - Apply toxidrome patterns to identify drug-induced syndromes. Anticholinergic toxidrome is characterized by CNS excitation (hallucinations and agitation), autonomic dysfunction (dryness and tachycardia), and urinary retention.
- *Early deprescribing*:
  - Discontinue offending medications immediately.
  - Focus on supportive care and symptomatic management to prevent complications.

Potential Harm from Unrecognized Adverse Drug Reactions

- *Delayed diagnosis and treatment:* Misattributing symptoms to disease progression may delay appropriate care, exacerbating patient morbidity.
- *Prescribing cascade*: Misdiagnosis may lead to unnecessary medications, compounding the risk of further ADRs. For instance, hallucinations in this case could lead to the initiation of antipsychotics, which carry risks of sedation, orthostatic hypotension, and extrapyramidal symptoms.
- *Healthcare burden:* ADRs contribute to prolonged hospital stays, increased diagnostic testing, and greater healthcare costs.

Management and Outcomes

Action Taken

Immediate discontinuation of promethazine: Identified as the key contributor to anticholinergic toxicity, promethazine was stopped.

Symptomatic Treatment

- Hydration with intravenous fluids improved systemic clearance of the drug.
- A short course of lorazepam was used to manage agitation without exacerbating anticholinergic effects.
- Urinary retention was managed with a temporary indwelling catheter.

Patient Education

- Counseling on the risks of self-medicating with over-the-counter drugs.
- Reinforcement of the importance of consulting healthcare providers before initiating new medications.

Systemic Changes

- The case was reported to pharmacovigilance authorities to highlight the risks associated with unsupervised use of over-the-counter anticholinergics.
- Institutional protocols were updated to include routine evaluation of anticholinergic burden in elderly patients.

Outcome

Patient recovery: Within 72 hours of intervention, Mrs ZB's symptoms resolved completely. She regained normal cognitive function and reported no lingering effects of toxicity.

Institutional Impact

Enhanced awareness and training on anticholinergic toxicity led to a reduction in ADR-related hospitalizations within the facility.

Discussion

This case underscores the importance of differentiating ADRs from disease progression in elderly patients. The overlap of symptoms can obscure the clinical picture, delaying accurate diagnosis and intervention.

In Mrs ZB's case, the additive effects of prescribed medications and an over-the-counter anticholinergic created a significant burden, manifesting as a toxidrome. Early recognition and intervention prevented further complications, highlighting the importance of a systematic approach to medication management.

Key lessons include:

- The necessity of regular medication reconciliation in elderly patients.
- The value of applying diagnostic frameworks like the toxidrome approach in complex presentations.
- The critical role of patient education in preventing self-medication-related harm.

BROADER IMPLICATIONS FOR PRACTICE

- *Promoting safe medication practices:* Educate patients and caregivers on the risks of self-medication and drug interactions.
- *Improving diagnostic accuracy:* Encourage clinicians to include ADRs in differential diagnoses, particularly when symptoms align with known drug effects.
- *Implementing institutional protocols:* Standardize the use of tools such as the ACB scale for evaluating anticholinergic load. Train staff to recognize and manage toxidromes effectively.
- *Strengthening pharmacovigilance:* Report ADR cases to national authorities to inform public health initiatives and guide regulatory decisions.

CONCLUSION

This case study illustrates the importance of recognizing ADRs as distinct from disease progression in elderly patients. Early identification of drug-induced conditions, informed by clinical frameworks and comprehensive medication reviews, ensures timely and effective management. For Mrs ZB, proactive measures not only resolved her symptoms but also underscored the value of vigilance in geriatric pharmacology. This approach exemplifies the broader goals of improving patient safety, optimizing therapeutic outcomes, and minimizing the societal burden of ADRs **(Box 1)**.

BOX 1 Key recommendations for clinical practice.

Avoid overprescription in asymptomatic conditions:

- *Guideline-adherent antibiotic use*: Refrain from prescribing antibiotics for asymptomatic bacteriuria (ASB) unless clear systemic or localized symptoms of infection are present
- *Routine screening*: Avoid routine urine cultures in asymptomatic elderly individuals to minimize unnecessary treatments and reduce antimicrobial resistance

Individualized renal function assessment:

- *Estimated glomerular filtration rate (eGFR)-based dosing*: Always calculate the eGFR using an appropriate formula (e.g., Cockcroft–Gault) to tailor dosing in elderly patients, especially for renally cleared drugs
- *Dynamic monitoring*: Regularly monitor renal function during treatment to adjust dosages based on acute changes

Recognize and manage adverse drug reactions:

- *Comprehensive medication reviews*: Assess for cumulative anticholinergic burden and polypharmacy risks during routine care
- *Early deprescribing*: Discontinue offending drugs promptly when adverse drug reactions (ADRs) are identified to prevent cascading complications

Promote antimicrobial and pharmacological stewardship:

- Educate healthcare providers and caregivers on the risks of overtreatment and self-medication
- Implement institutional protocols to standardize evidence-based prescribing practices

Enhance diagnostic accuracy:

- Use diagnostic frameworks, such as toxidrome recognition, to distinguish ADRs from disease progression
- Prioritize patient-specific evaluations to prevent misdiagnosis and unnecessary interventions

Patient-centered approach in elderly care:

- *Education and counseling*: Empower patients and families to understand the risks and benefits of treatment decisions, fostering shared decision-making
- *Fostering vigilance*: Encourage regular follow-ups and proactive communication about medication side effects

Institutional policy recommendations:

- Standardize use of the Anticholinergic Cognitive Burden (ACB) scale and other tools for assessing medication risks
- Implement multidisciplinary medication reconciliation teams to review complex cases
- Report ADRs to pharmacovigilance systems to contribute to broader public health data

Note: By integrating these recommendations, healthcare providers can ensure safer, evidence-based management of elderly patients, reducing the risks of adverse outcomes and supporting a culture of rational prescribing.

SUGGESTED READINGS

1. Nicolle LE, Gupta K, Bradley SF, Colgan R, DeMuri GP, Drekonja D, et al. Clinical Practice Guideline for the Management of Asymptomatic Bacteriuria: 2019 Update by the Infectious Diseases Society of America. Clin Infect Dis. 2019;68(10):e83-e110.
2. Samajdar SS, Sharma J, Mukherjee S, Sahoo S, Sarkar S, Pal J, et al. Clinical Pharmacological Principles in Emergency Geriatric Care: Toxidrome Approach. J Indian Acad Geriatr. 2023;19(4):282-4.
3. Samajdar SS, Mukherjee S, Sarkar S, Chatterjee N, Roy MK, Pal J, et al. Prescribing Cascade Complicating a Geriatric Patient. J Indian Acad Geriatr. 2024;20(1):40-2.

9

CHAPTER

Conclusion and Future Directions

ABSTRACT

Transforming Elderly Care for a Better Tomorrow

The concluding chapter synthesizes the evolving landscape of elderly care, emphasizing the critical need for integrated, patient-centered, and evidence-based approaches to address the multifaceted challenges of aging populations. Key takeaways highlight the importance of rational prescribing, considering age-related physiological changes, polypharmacy management, and deprescribing, supported by tools such as the Beers Criteria and STOPP/START frameworks. The adoption of the Integrated Care for Older People (ICOPE) framework provides a unified methodology for promoting functional independence, while leveraging non-pharmacological interventions and personalized medicine ensures holistic well-being. Future directions include the integration of artificial intelligence (AI) for predictive insights, precision medicine for tailored treatments, and global collaboration to share best practices and address disparities. Advancements in healthcare delivery models, such as telemedicine, home-based care, and community-driven support, offer scalable solutions to meet the growing demands. By fostering interdisciplinary communication and leveraging emerging technologies, healthcare systems can create sustainable, equitable, and impactful elderly care strategies for a healthier tomorrow.

A dedicated section highlights the importance of systematized prescribing practices tailored to India's geriatric care needs, encapsulated in **Table 1**, which categorizes medications based on therapeutic systems, specific drugs available in India, their indications, considerations for elderly patients, and safer alternatives. By addressing key challenges such as polypharmacy, drug interactions, and age-related changes in pharmacokinetics, the table serves as a practical guideline for clinicians. Its evidence-based recommendations integrate international frameworks such as the BEERS Criteria while accommodating local drug availability and healthcare infrastructure, emphasizing safer pharmacotherapy practices for India's aging population.

TABLE 1: Indian guidelines for rational prescribing in elderly care.

System	Drug class	Drugs available in India	Indication/Use	Specific considerations for elderly	Alternatives (if any)
Central nervous	Benzodiazepines	Diazepam, lorazepam, and clonazepam	Anxiety and insomnia	Risk of falls, sedation; short-term use only	CBT or short-term Z-drugs like zolpidem
	Antidepressants	Amitriptyline, sertraline, and escitalopram	Depression	Avoid TCAs like amitriptyline in cardiac/orthostatic issues; prefer SSRIs	Escitalopram and sertraline
	Antiepileptics	Phenytoin, levetiracetam, and gabapentin	Seizures, neuropathic pain	Monitor sedation and renal function; gabapentin risk of dependence	Levetiracetam
	Antipsychotics	Haloperidol, risperidone, and olanzapine	Psychosis, agitation in dementia	Risk of stroke, sedation; use the lowest effective dose	Behavioral therapy
Cardiovascular	Antihypertensives	Amlodipine, telmisartan, and losartan	Hypertension	Avoid beta-blockers in bradycardia; monitor electrolytes with diuretics	ARBs like telmisartan
	Beta-blockers	Atenolol, bisoprolol. and nebivolol	Hypertension and arrhythmias	Risk of bradycardia; avoid abrupt withdrawal	Bisoprolol
	Diuretics	Furosemide, spironolactone, and torsemide	Heart failure, edema	Electrolyte imbalances; avoid in severe renal failure	Torsemide
	Anticoagulants	Warfarin, apixaban, dabigatran	Atrial fibrillation, stroke prevention	Monitor INR for warfarin; increased bleeding risk	Apixaban preferred
Endocrine	Oral hypoglycemics	Metformin, glimepiride, and dapagliflozin	Type 2 diabetes	Risk of hypoglycemia with sulfonylureas; monitor renal function	DPP-4 inhibitors like sitagliptin
	Insulins	Regular insulin, glargine, and lispro	Type 1 and type 2 diabetes	Tailor regimen to avoid hypoglycemia; consider pre-mixed insulins	Basal insulins (e.g., glargine)
	Thyroid hormones	Levothyroxine	Hypothyroidism	Monitor TSH levels regularly	None

Continued

Continued

System	Drug class	Drugs available in India	Indication/Use	Specific considerations for elderly	Alternatives (if any)
Respiratory	Bronchodilators	Salbutamol, tiotropium, and formoterol	Asthma and COPD	Monitor tachycardia with beta-agonists; avoid overuse of short-acting inhalers	Tiotropium (long-acting)
	Corticosteroids (inhaled)	Budesonide and fluticasone	Asthma, COPD	Long-term use may increase osteoporosis risk	Low-dose inhaled preferred
Gastrointestinal	Proton pump inhibitors (PPIs)	Pantoprazole and omeprazole, esomeprazole	GERD and peptic ulcer disease	Long-term use risks fractures and infections	H2-blockers like ranitidine
	Laxatives	Lactulose, polyethylene glycol, and psyllium	Constipation	Avoid stimulant laxatives for chronic use	Bulk-forming agents
Musculoskeletal	NSAIDs	Ibuprofen, diclofenac, and naproxen	Pain, inflammation	Risk of GI bleeding, renal impairment; avoid in ulcer disease	Paracetamol (preferred)
	DMARDs	Methotrexate, hydroxychloroquine, and sulfasalazine	Rheumatoid arthritis	Monitor for hepatotoxicity, retinal damage (hydroxychloroquine)	Biologics (if available)
Infectious diseases	Antibiotics	Amoxicillin, azithromycin, and ciprofloxacin	Bacterial infections	Adjust dose in renal failure; monitor for resistance	Doxycycline
	Antifungals	Fluconazole, itraconazole, and voriconazole	Fungal infections	Monitor hepatic function	Terbinafine
	Antivirals	Acyclovir and oseltamivir	Herpes simplex and influenza	Monitor renal function for acyclovir	Oseltamivir for influenza
Urinary	Anticholinergics	Oxybutynin and tolterodine	Overactive bladder	Avoid in dementia or cognitive impairment due to anticholinergic burden	Mirabegron (it increases in blood pressure—monitor BP)
	Alpha-blockers	Tamsulosin, alfuzosin, and silodosin	Benign prostatic hyperplasia	Risk of orthostatic hypotension; start with a low dose	Silodosin

INTRODUCTION

Elderly care stands at the crossroads of opportunity and challenge, shaped by the rapid aging of populations, breakthroughs in medicine, and the intricate demands of geriatric pharmacotherapy. This final chapter synthesizes the key takeaways from the preceding discussions and provides a roadmap for addressing the unique and evolving needs of older adults.

The solutions lie in adopting an integrated, evidence-based, and patient-centered approach to healthcare. By advancing rational prescribing practices, leveraging technology, and fostering collaboration among stakeholders, the future of elderly care can be transformed into a sustainable, inclusive, and effective system.

The chapter explores actionable recommendations, highlights innovations such as the Integrated Care for Older People (ICOPE) framework and remote patient monitoring (RPM), and delves into future directions, including artificial intelligence, precision medicine, and holistic care models. These strategies will ensure that the aging population receives not only the best possible medical interventions but also a holistic approach to well-being that embraces psychological, social, and environmental factors.

KEY TAKEAWAYS

- *Rational prescribing as a cornerstone of geriatric care*:
  - Safe and effective medication use for elderly patients requires adherence to rational prescribing principles, including patient-centered care, evidence-based practice, and shared decision-making.
  - The *5R* framework (*r*ight drug, *r*ight dose, *r*ight route, *r*ight duration, and *r*ight monitoring) provides a structured approach to achieving optimal outcomes.
- *Age-related physiological changes impact medication use*:
  - Pharmacokinetic and pharmacodynamic changes in aging significantly influence drug absorption, metabolism, and excretion.
  - These changes necessitate tailored drug selection, dosage adjustments, and vigilant monitoring to minimize adverse drug reactions (ADRs).
- *Polypharmacy and deprescribing are central challenges*:
  - Polypharmacy increases risks of ADRs, drug-drug interactions, and non-adherence.
  - Deprescribing, guided by tools such as the Beers Criteria and screening tool of older people's prescriptions (STOPP)/screening tool to alert to right treatment (START) frameworks, is crucial to reducing medication burden while maintaining therapeutic efficacy.
- *The role of non-pharmacological interventions:*
  - Non-drug therapies, such as cognitive-behavioral therapy for insomnia (CBT-I) and physical activity, provide effective alternatives to pharmacological treatments.
  - These interventions address the holistic needs of elderly patients and reduce dependency on medications.

- *Ethical and legal considerations are fundamental:*
    - Informed consent, respect for autonomy, and shared decision-making are vital to ethical prescribing.
    - Legal frameworks ensure adherence to guidelines and protect patient rights, especially in cases of cognitive impairment or end-of-life care.
- *Personalized medicine is the future of elderly care:*
    - Pharmacogenomics and caregiver involvement enhance medication management by aligning treatments with individual genetic, social, and clinical profiles.
    - Personalized approaches improve therapeutic outcomes and reduce healthcare disparities.
- *Guidelines for rational prescribing: Focus on the Indian context:* **Table 1** provides a comprehensive guideline for rational prescribing in elderly care, tailored to the Indian context. It categorizes medications system-wise, including their drug classes, examples of drugs available in India, primary indications, specific considerations for elderly patients, and safer alternatives where applicable. Highlighting key geriatric challenges such as polypharmacy, drug-drug interactions, and age-related physiological changes, the table emphasizes the need for caution with medications such as benzodiazepines, non-steroidal anti-inflammatory drugs (NSAIDs), and anticholinergics due to their potential for adverse effects. It also promotes the use of safer options, such as selective serotonin reuptake inhibitors (SSRIs) over tricyclic antidepressants (TCAs) for depression or paracetamol over NSAIDs for pain management. This evidence-based approach aligns with global guidelines such as the BEERS criteria while addressing the unique availability and affordability of medications in India, ensuring effective and safe geriatric pharmacotherapy.

INTEGRATED CARE FOR OLDER PEOPLE: A FRAMEWORK FOR HOLISTIC ELDERLY CARE

The ICOPE framework, developed by the World Health Organization (WHO), offers a comprehensive, person-centered approach to managing the health and well-being of older adults. This model emphasizes early detection, prevention, and management of declines in intrinsic capacity through integrated, evidence-based interventions. Below is a dedicated section on ICOPE to be incorporated into the conclusion chapter, reflecting its importance in the broader context of rational prescribing and elderly care.

INTEGRATED CARE FOR OLDER PEOPLE: A UNIFIED APPROACH TO ELDERLY CARE

As global populations age, healthcare systems face increasing challenges in addressing the multidimensional needs of older adults. The ICOPE guidelines provide a structured methodology to prevent, delay, or reverse declines in physical, cognitive, and emotional capacities, ensuring that older individuals maintain their functional independence and quality of life.

KEY COMPONENTS OF THE INTEGRATED CARE FOR OLDER PEOPLE FRAMEWORK

- *Comprehensive assessment and integrated care planning:*
  - Older adults are evaluated for declines in mobility, nutrition, cognition, vision, hearing, and emotional well-being.
  - A unified care plan integrates interventions across all domains to address interconnected health issues holistically.
- *Evidence-based interventions:*
  - *Mobility:* Multimodal exercise programs combining resistance, balance, flexibility, and aerobic training improve mobility and reduce fall risks.
  - *Nutrition:* Dietary counseling and oral nutritional supplementation address undernutrition, sarcopenia, and related conditions.
  - *Vision and hearing:* Routine screenings and timely provision of eyeglasses or hearing aids restore sensory capacities and reduce isolation.
  - *Cognition:* Cognitive stimulation therapies help maintain or improve cognitive function, particularly in those at risk of dementia.
  - *Mental health:* Structured psychological interventions and physical activity are recommended to manage depressive symptoms.
- *Addressing geriatric syndromes*:
  - *Urinary incontinence:* Pelvic floor muscle training and bladder control strategies improve continence and reduce care dependency.
  - *Falls prevention:* Multifactorial interventions, including medication reviews and home modifications, mitigate fall risks.
- *Caregiver support:* Psychological interventions, skill-building, and respite care for caregivers alleviate strain and ensure sustainable caregiving practices.

KEY RECOMMENDATIONS FOR IMPLEMENTATION

- Integrated care delivery
- Integrated care for older people encourages a person-centered approach where all interventions are combined to address multiple health issues simultaneously, ensuring efficiency and improved outcomes.
- *Early detection and tailored interventions:* Impairments in intrinsic capacity trigger timely medical evaluations and individualized care plans.
- *Community-based implementation:* The framework prioritizes task-shifting to community health workers and family caregivers, ensuring accessibility in low-resource settings.
- *Policy integration:* Policymakers must incorporate ICOPE principles into national health strategies to address the growing demands of aging populations.

FUTURE DIRECTIONS FOR INTEGRATED CARE FOR OLDER PEOPLE INTEGRATION

Scaling Up Interventions

- Expand access to ICOPE-recommended programs through telemedicine and mobile health units.
- Develop training programs for community health workers to deliver care at the grassroots level.

Strengthening Research

- Conduct studies on the long-term impacts of ICOPE interventions, particularly in low- and middle-income countries.
- Explore innovative models combining ICOPE with digital health solutions.

Global Collaboration

Facilitate knowledge-sharing initiatives to align global health systems with the ICOPE framework.

Enhancing Equity

Address healthcare disparities by prioritizing underserved populations in ICOPE implementation plans.

The ICOPE framework underscores the importance of integrated, patient-centered, and preventive care for older adults. By embedding these principles into geriatric healthcare systems, the global community can ensure healthier aging and improve the overall quality of life for older populations.

OUR RECOMMENDATIONS FOR IMPROVING ELDERLY CARE

- *Strengthen geriatric clinical pharmacology education:*
    - Incorporate geriatric clinical pharmacology and rational prescribing modules into medical and nursing curricula.
    - Provide ongoing training on tools such as STOPP/START, Beers Criteria, and deprescribing algorithms.
- *Promote multidisciplinary collaboration:*
    - Establish care teams comprising physicians, pharmacists, nurses, and caregivers to ensure holistic patient management.
    - Encourage collaboration between specialties to address comorbidities and optimize medication regimens.
- *Leverage technology for safer prescribing:*
    - Integrate electronic health records (EHRs) with clinical decision-support systems (CDSS) to flag potentially inappropriate medications (PIMs) and drug-drug interactions (DDIs).
    - Develop mobile apps for easy access to prescribing guidelines and patient-specific tools.

- *Enhance access to non-pharmacological interventions:*
  - Increase awareness and availability of evidence-based therapies such as CBT-I, mindfulness, and physical activity programs.
  - Subsidize non-drug therapies to make them accessible to marginalized populations.
- *Implement comprehensive medication review programs:*
  - Conduct regular medication reviews in primary care, hospital settings, and long-term care facilities.
  - Use structured frameworks such as medication therapy management (MTM) and comprehensive medication reviews (CMRs) to identify and mitigate risks.
- *Encourage policy and regulatory reforms:*
  - Advocate for policies promoting the use of generics, deprescribing initiatives, and rational prescribing frameworks.
  - Establish monitoring systems for ADRs and DDIs, especially in vulnerable elderly populations.
- *Focus on patient and caregiver empowerment:*
  - Educate elderly patients and their families about medication management, ADRs, and the importance of adherence.
  - Develop culturally sensitive materials and resources to support informed decision-making.
- *Advance research in geriatric pharmacotherapy:*
  - Encourage clinical trials involving older adults to generate robust evidence for prescribing guidelines.
  - Prioritize research on emerging fields such as pharmacogenomics, drug-disease interactions, and non-pharmacological therapies.
- *Adopt a patient-centered approach to elderly care:*
  - Align treatment plans with the values, preferences, and goals of elderly patients.
  - Ensure continuity of care through effective communication between healthcare providers and patients.
- *Strengthen adverse drug reaction reporting systems:*
  - Train healthcare providers on the importance of ADR reporting and the use of pharmacovigilance platforms.
  - Simplify reporting mechanisms to encourage higher participation.

INTEGRATING REMOTE PATIENT MONITORING INTO ELDERLY CARE

The incorporation of RPM technologies has significantly enhanced clinicians' ability to monitor and manage patients beyond traditional healthcare settings. By leveraging noninvasive digital tools, RPM facilitates the continuous collection and transmission of health data from patients' homes to healthcare providers, enabling timely interventions and improved healthcare decision-making. This approach aligns seamlessly with our recommendations for improving elderly care, offering a transformative opportunity to enhance safety, efficiency, and personalization in geriatric medicine.

BENEFITS OF REMOTE PATIENT MONITORING FOR ELDERLY CARE

- Improved access and continuity of care
- Remote patient monitoring bridges the gap between patients and healthcare providers, allowing real-time monitoring of vital signs such as blood pressure, oxygen levels, heart rate, and weight.
  - Chronic conditions such as diabetes, hypertension, and heart failure can be managed more effectively by integrating RPM into routine care plans.
- *Facilitation of clinical pharmacological reconciliation review and feedback (CPRRF)*
  - Remote patient monitoring provides continuous data streams, enabling clinical pharmacologists and geriatricians to review medication effectiveness, adherence, and potential ADRs.
  - Clinical pharmacological reconciliation review and feedback through RPM ensures timely adjustments to medication regimens, particularly in polypharmacy scenarios common among older adults.
- *Enhanced multidisciplinary collaboration:*
  - Data from RPM can be shared among multidisciplinary teams, including geriatricians, internal medicine experts, clinical pharmacologists, pharmacists, and nurses, to develop and adjust integrated care plans.
  - By providing centralized access to patient health metrics, RPM fosters better communication and coordination among care teams.
- *Empowerment of patients and caregivers:*
  - Wearable devices and user-friendly interfaces empower elderly patients to engage with their health actively.
  - Caregivers benefit from real-time updates, easing the burden of constant oversight and enabling timely interventions. Tools such as pill reminders and recording functionalities on mobile applications enhance convenience and support medication adherence, promoting better compliance with prescribed treatments.

RECOMMENDATIONS FOR REMOTE PATIENT MONITORING IMPLEMENTATION IN ELDERLY CARE

- *Leverage RPM in geriatric clinical pharmacology:* Integrate RPM training into geriatric clinical pharmacology education, enabling clinicians to interpret RPM data for safer prescribing and deprescribing practices.
- *Enhance medication safety with remote patient monitoring:*
  - Combine RPM data with EHRs and CDSS to flag PIMs and monitor DDIs.
- *Promote personalized and preventive medicine:*
  - Utilize RPM to tailor treatment plans based on individual health trends and risk factors.
  - Develop predictive analytics tools to preempt complications such as falls or acute exacerbations of chronic conditions.

- *Expand access to remote patient monitoring technologies:*
    - Provide subsidies or incentives to ensure the affordability of RPM devices for elderly populations, especially in underserved areas.
    - Train community health workers to support RPM deployment and troubleshooting for older adults with limited technological literacy.
- *Foster research and policy support:*
    - Encourage studies on the long-term benefits of RPM in reducing hospitalizations and healthcare costs in geriatric populations.
    - Advocate for policies that promote the integration of RPM into standard elderly care frameworks, ensuring equitable access and reimbursement.

FUTURE DIRECTIONS FOR REMOTE PATIENT MONITORING IN ELDERLY CARE

- *Artificial intelligence-driven insights from remote patient monitoring data:* Leverage artificial intelligence to analyze RPM data for detecting early warning signs of clinical deterioration, thereby enhancing preventive care. Establishing a robust, organized repository of RPM data from diverse centers across India can facilitate the development of uniform healthcare policies, embodying the concept of Big Data to drive systemic improvements and informed decision-making.
- *Integration with non-pharmacological interventions:* Combine RPM with digital platforms for guided physical therapy, cognitive stimulation, and mindfulness exercises tailored for elderly users.
- *Culturally adapted remote patient monitoring solutions:* Develop RPM interfaces and educational materials tailored to the diverse linguistic and cultural needs of elderly populations. Incorporating on-the-spot, recognized-registered language options or single-click translations with subtitles can significantly enhance accessibility and user engagement, ensuring inclusivity across different demographic groups.

By embedding RPM technologies into geriatric care, healthcare systems can significantly enhance patient outcomes, reduce hospital readmissions, and empower elderly individuals to lead healthier, more independent lives. Positioned as a cornerstone of modern elderly care, RPM ensures that clinicians remain connected to their patients, offering timely, data-driven, and personalized interventions.

FUTURE DIRECTIONS IN ELDERLY CARE

The future of elderly care demands a proactive, innovative, and patient-centered approach to address the growing complexities of aging populations. Key advancements in technology, healthcare delivery, and international collaboration will shape the landscape of geriatric care, ensuring sustainable and equitable solutions. Below is an elaboration of critical future directions for improving elderly care.

Integration of Artificial Intelligence in Geriatric Care

Artificial intelligence holds transformative potential in the field of elderly care by enhancing predictive, diagnostic, and therapeutic capabilities.

- *Identifying high-risk patients:* AI algorithms can analyze large datasets, including health records and RPM data, to identify early warning signs of conditions such as frailty, cognitive decline, or acute exacerbations of chronic diseases.
- *Predicting ADRs:* Machine learning models can predict ADRs by evaluating patient-specific factors, drug interactions, and genetic predispositions, thereby supporting safer prescribing practices.
- *Optimizing medication regimens:* AI-powered tools can recommend personalized medication adjustments based on real-time health data and clinical guidelines, improving treatment efficacy and adherence.
- *Enhancing care efficiency:* AI-enabled virtual assistants and chatbots can assist with routine tasks such as appointment scheduling, medication reminders, and patient education, reducing the burden on caregivers and healthcare providers.

Expansion of Precision Medicine

Precision medicine focuses on tailoring medical treatments to individual characteristics, including genetic, environmental, and lifestyle factors.

- *Pharmacogenomics in geriatric care:* Advances in pharmacogenomics will enable clinicians to predict how older adults metabolize specific drugs, reducing the risk of ADRs and optimizing drug selection and dosing.
- *Targeted therapies:* Precision medicine can offer targeted interventions for age-related conditions such as cancer, cardiovascular diseases, and neurodegenerative disorders, enhancing therapeutic outcomes.
- *Personalized prevention:* Genetic screening and biomarker analysis can help identify predispositions to diseases, allowing early intervention and prevention strategies customized to individual needs.

Holistic Care Models

The aging process is multifaceted, encompassing physical, psychological, social, and environmental dimensions that require integrated care models.

- *Multidimensional assessments:* Future care models will incorporate comprehensive assessments that address not just medical but also social determinants of health, such as living conditions, financial status, and social support networks.
- *Integrated interventions:* Holistic care plans will combine medical treatments with non-pharmacological interventions such as physical therapy, cognitive stimulation, and mental health counseling to address the diverse needs of elderly patients.
- *Community-based support:* Programs emphasizing social engagement, community participation, and caregiver education will enhance the overall quality of life for older adults and reduce care dependency.

Global Collaboration

International cooperation is critical to addressing the challenges posed by aging populations worldwide.

- *Sharing best practices:* Collaborative efforts between countries can help develop and disseminate effective models of elderly care, ensuring that successful interventions are adapted to diverse cultural and economic contexts.
- *Data integration and standardization:* Cross-border sharing of anonymized health data can facilitate large-scale research on aging, enabling the development of universally applicable guidelines and benchmarks.
- *Capacity building:* Training programs and knowledge-sharing initiatives can empower healthcare professionals in low- and middle-income countries to provide high-quality geriatric care.
- *Global health policies:* International organizations, such as the WHO, can play a pivotal role in advocating for policies that prioritize elderly care and promote equity in resource allocation.

Innovative Healthcare Delivery Models

Advancements in technology and service delivery methods will redefine how care is provided to elderly populations, particularly in underserved areas.

- *Telemedicine:* Virtual consultations will expand access to specialists for elderly patients in remote locations, reducing travel-related challenges and improving continuity of care.
- *Mobile health units:* These units can deliver comprehensive geriatric services, including screenings, medication reviews, and vaccinations, directly to communities with limited healthcare infrastructure.
- *Home-based care models:* RPM and in-home health services will support aging in place, enabling elderly individuals to receive care in familiar and comfortable settings.
- *Task shifting and training:* Equipping non-specialist health workers and caregivers with the tools and training to provide basic geriatric care will alleviate workforce shortages and enhance care accessibility.
- *Foster broad interdisciplinary communication and collaboration* among stakeholders in technology, AI, and medical device fields by establishing integrated forums, workshops, and networks. These platforms should focus on sharing specific needs, challenges, and innovations to bridge knowledge gaps, identify synergies, and accelerate the development of impactful, cross-disciplinary solutions.

CONCLUSION

This chapter underscores the importance of adopting integrated, patient-centered approaches in elderly care to address the multifaceted challenges of aging populations. It emphasizes the significance of rational prescribing, deprescribing, and leveraging innovative frameworks like the Integrated Care for Older People (ICOPE) to promote functional independence and holistic well-being. By integrating evidence-based practices with non-pharmacological interventions and emerging technologies, healthcare systems can address the complexities of geriatric care, ensuring equitable and sustainable outcomes. For practical application, detailed algorithms and flowcharts in the Appendix provide step-by-step guidance on deprescribing, enhancing safety and effectiveness in medication management tailored to the Indian healthcare context.

SUGGESTED READINGS

1. Integrated Care for Older People: Guidelines on Community-Level Interventions to Manage Declines in Intrinsic Capacity. Geneva: World Health Organization; 2017. 3, Evidence and recommendations.
2. Vegesna A, Tran M, Angelaccio M, Arcona S. Remote Patient Monitoring via Non-Invasive Digital Technologies: A Systematic Review. Telemed J E Health. 2017;23(1):3-17.
3. LeadingAge CAST. Telehealth and Remote Patient Monitoring for Long Term and Post Acute Care: A Primer and Provider Selection Guide 2015. Washington, DC: LeadingAge Center for Aging Services Technologies; 2015.
4. Tan SY, Sumner J, Wang Y, Wenjun Yip A. A systematic review of the impacts of remote patient monitoring (RPM) interventions on safety, adherence, quality-of-life and cost-related outcomes. NPJ Digit Med. 2024;7(1):192.

APPENDIX

APPENDIX A: DETAILED ALGORITHMS AND FLOWCHARTS FOR THE DEPRESCRIBING PROCESS (ALGORITHM 1)

This appendix provides a comprehensive framework for the deprescribing process, customized for the Indian healthcare context. It includes step-by-step algorithms and flowcharts that address common medications, prevalent conditions, and cultural practices to guide healthcare providers in rationalizing medication use for elderly patients.

Algorithm 1: Deprescribing Process Overview

Ascertain All Medications

- Compile a complete list of the patient's medications, including prescribed drugs, over-the-counter products, and traditional remedies commonly used in India.
- Assess adherence patterns and identify any polypharmacy practices.

Identify High-risk Medications

Focus on drugs with high anticholinergic burden, sedatives, nonsteroidal anti-inflammatory drugs (NSAIDs), and long-term proton pump inhibitors (PPIs), as these are frequently implicated in adverse reactions among Indian populations.

Evaluate Patient-specific Risks and Benefits

- Use risk prediction tools adapted to Indian demographic and health data.
- Consider factors such as age, comorbidities, renal function, and sociocultural influences.

Classify Medications Using a Utility Grid

- *Class A:* Very effective, minimal toxicity (e.g., melatonin as sedative in elderly).
- *Class B:* Reasonable efficacy, some toxicity concerns (e.g., NSAIDs with gastrointestinal risks).
- *Class C:* Effectiveness and toxicity concerns (e.g., barbiturate as sedatives in elderly patients).
- *Class D:* Minimal effectiveness, high toxicity potential (e.g., PPIs without clear indications).

Engage Patients and Families in Shared Decision-making

- Conduct respectful and culturally aware discussions to explain the rationale for deprescribing.
- Address patient concerns and involve family members to build trust and ensure adherence.

Implement and Monitor

- Gradually taper or stop medications as appropriate.
- Schedule follow-ups to monitor for withdrawal symptoms and evaluate therapeutic outcomes.

APPENDIX B: EDUCATIONAL MATERIALS AND PATIENT INFORMATION LEAFLETS

This appendix includes educational resources aimed at enhancing patient understanding of the deprescribing process. Materials are culturally adapted, accessible in multiple Indian languages, and designed to engage both patients and their families.

Patient Leaflet 1: Understanding Deprescribing

- *Content:* An easy-to-understand explanation of deprescribing, its role in reducing unnecessary medications, and its benefits in improving health outcomes.
- *Target audience:* Elderly patients and their caregivers.
- *Cultural relevance:* It includes relatable examples of commonly deprescribed medications in India, such as NSAIDs and sedatives.

Patient Leaflet 2: Managing Common Withdrawal Symptoms

- *Content:* Practical advice for recognizing and managing withdrawal symptoms associated with specific drug classes (e.g., sedatives, antihypertensives).
- *Tips:*
    - How to manage insomnia during benzodiazepine withdrawal.
    - Dietary and lifestyle modifications for rebound acidity after discontinuing PPIs.

Patient Leaflet 3: Family Support in Deprescribing

- *Content:* Guidance for family members to provide emotional and practical support to elderly patients undergoing medication changes.
- *Focus:* Strategies for encouraging adherence, monitoring for side effects, and seeking medical help if necessary.

TABLE SUMMARIES

Table 2 highlights key strategies for effectively engaging patients in the deprescribing process, emphasizing culturally tailored communication, family involvement, and the use of visual aids. These strategies are designed to foster understanding, trust, and collaboration, which are essential for successful deprescribing initiatives. **Table 3** focuses on managing withdrawal symptoms associated with deprescribing specific drug classes, such as benzodiazepines, proton pump inhibitors (PPIs), and NSAIDs. It provides practical management tips, including gradual tapering, dietary adjustments, and the use of alternative therapies, ensuring patient comfort and minimizing adverse effects during the transition. Together, these tables offer a structured framework to support healthcare providers in addressing the complexities of deprescribing while prioritizing patient-centered care.

TABLE 2: Key strategies for patient engagement.

Strategy	Description
Culturally tailored communication	Use local languages, metaphors, and examples to explain deprescribing benefits
Family involvement	Involve family members in discussions to foster trust and shared decision-making
Visual aids	Employ charts, diagrams, and flowcharts to simplify complex information for patients and caregivers

TABLE 3: Managing withdrawal symptoms.

Drug class	Common withdrawal symptoms	Management tips
Benzodiazepines	Insomnia and anxiety	Gradual tapering, use of non-pharmacological therapies like CBT
PPIs	Rebound acidity	Dietary modifications, short-term use of H2-blockers
NSAIDs	Increased pain perception	Switch to paracetamol, consider physiotherapy for pain management

These appendices provide actionable tools and culturally sensitive resources for implementing deprescribing initiatives in the Indian healthcare setting. By addressing both clinical and patient-centered aspects, they aim to enhance the safety, efficacy, and acceptance of deprescribing practices, ultimately contributing to better health outcomes for elderly patients.

Index

Page numbers followed by *b* refer to box and *t* refer to table.

A

H

I